The Frontal Brain
and Language

The Frontal Brain and Language

Edison K. Miyawaki, M.D.

Copyright © 2018 by Edison K. Miyawaki, M.D.

Library of Congress Control Number: 2018909713
ISBN: Hardcover 978-1-9845-4788-0
Softcover 978-1-9845-4790-3
eBook 978-1-9845-4789-7

All rights reserved. No part of this book may be reproduced or transmitted in any form or by any means, electronic or mechanical, including photocopying, recording, or by any information storage and retrieval system, without permission in writing from the copyright owner.

Any people depicted in stock imagery provided by Getty Images are models, and such images are being used for illustrative purposes only.
Certain stock imagery © Getty Images.

Print information available on the last page.

Rev. date: 08/16/2018

To order additional copies of this book, contact:
Xlibris
1-888-795-4274
www.Xlibris.com
Orders@Xlibris.com

Contents

1. Foreword..1
2. London, around 1860 2
3. Paris, 1861-1865 10
4. Breslau and Vienna, 1874.......................................15
5. Leipzig, 1898 23
6. Sound 27
7. Arrival at Primary Auditory Cortex........................33
8. Pierre Marie's Issue..39
9. A Problem With Naming, Part I............................43
10. A Problem With Naming, Part II...........................50
11. Frontal Sparing?..55
12. Connectivity I: Hodology 61
13. Connectivity II: Projection and Association 67
14. Connectivity III: An Old Paper 72
15. A Note on Dominance..77
16. Metaconnectivity 81
17. Historical and Contemporary Conclusion.............89

References 91

1.

Foreword

Our big story, made up of little ones, starts in London, England. The year is 1860, give or take. We'll end with the present day.

Like my previous short book, *The Crossed Organization of Brains*, this monograph is intended for the interested medical or neuroscience student.

Chapters two through five cover some history of brain science.

Then we'll talk about what Shakespeare's Hamlet called "words, words, words."

2.

London, around 1860

Europeans, especially the British, sometimes double up their last names. If your mom's family's name is "Hughlings" and your dad's family name is "Jackson," you end up being a "Hughlings Jackson." In scientific publications, you'll find references to Jackson, J. H. rather than Hughlings Jackson, J. It's a little confusing. I'll call him John.

John married a woman named Elizabeth Dade.

We'll get to her in a moment.

In 1859, when John was 24 years old, he moved from the northern English countryside to London to continue his medical education. In the capital, people were abuzz about a new book, *On the Origin of Species*. Of course you've heard about it, even if you've never read a word by Charles Darwin. Likewise, many Londoners knew about the idea of evolution by hearsay.

John attended hospital conferences and reported for a magazine called the *Medical Times and Gazette*. He wrote about patients with various brain problems–some with neurosyphilis, some with seizures, some with both. I don't know for a fact when John witnessed his first seizure as a clinician.

I do know for a fact that Elizabeth Dade Jackson, whom John married in 1865, eventually had the kind of seizure that we now call "Jacksonian." She died in 1876, and people say John never got over it.

John is also associated with evolutionary theory.

Seizures *and* the origin of species: what do these have to do with one another? Let's start with the seizures.

John's namesake type of seizure, first of all, has to do with the frontal brain.

It turns out that a Jacksonian seizure had been described decades before, by a Frenchman named Bravais. John knew about Bravais; he didn't plagiarize. But we don't talk about Bravaisian seizures today.

In seizures of the Jacksonian type, you might see a big toe jerk rhythmically, then the foot and the toes, then the leg and the foot and toes, then the arm right down to the fingers (along with the whole leg), then the face along with everything else, just on one side of the body. Even as the sequence transpires, the person could be awake and even talking. John could look at a case of a jerking right thumb with a tumor the size of a hazelnut in the left frontal cortex, and he couldn't help but think that the front of the brain was involved in movement.

Around 1860, textbooks taught that the cerebral cortex didn't control movement. In Italy, circa 1810, Luigi Rolando irritated cortex and he noticed movements on the opposite side of the body. His experiments were roundly criticized. His reviewers said that stimulation at the brain's surface passed through to deeper areas. His was no proof for a role for cortex in the generation of movement, they said.

Does it seem odd to you that the subcortex alone could drive movement—or that people once believed so? From 1810 to 1860, experimenters poked at the cortical surface or just beneath it, but they didn't learn much. Here is François Achelle Longet, of Paris, writing in the 19th century: "On dogs, rabbits and on some kids we have irritated with a knife the white substance of the cerebral lobes, we have cauterised them with potash, nitric acid, etc.; we have run galvanic currents through them in all directions without succeeding in evoking involuntary muscular contractions; the same negative results were found in directing these agents to either gray or white matter" (quoted in McHenry, 1969). "Kids" refers to goats.

*

Enter a man named Charles E. Brown, who was 43 years old in 1860. His dad was a sea captain from Philadelphia; his mom was French. When he finished medical school in Paris, Charles wanted a more unusual name than "Brown," so he added his mom's last name to his dad's. He became Charles E. Brown-Séquard (Aminoff, 1993).

He ran a place called the National Hospital in London, beginning in 1860. The National Hospital still exists today, but, at that time, it had just opened in a donated townhouse. Its infirmary had eight beds; there were some consulting rooms for outpatients; the pharmacy was a butler's pantry.

Brown-Séquard brought a new French school of thought about the brain to London. The French perspective held that the frontal brain had to do with speech and language. Brown-Séquard hired John as an assistant at the National Hospital.

To get more of a sense of the French school, let's think about a patient discussed in Paris on April 4, 1861. I don't know the patient's name, but the doctor was Ernest Auburtin.

Auburtin described how his patient had shot himself at the head in an attempted suicide. That would be "at," not "in" the head. The attempted suicide wasn't successful, not at first. The shot glanced, sheared away the front of the skull, but left the underlying brain intact.

Auburtin said that the man's intelligence and speech were normal after the accident.

The patient could speak reasonably enough and was reportedly normal aside from his missing frontal skull. The brain was visible. Auburtin did an odd thing with a spatula–seriously, a spatula. He pressed on the exposed brain: "While the patient was being interrogated the flat surface of a large spatula was lightly applied; on gentle pressure speech was suddenly suspended; a word begun was cut in two. Speech returned as soon as pressure was removed. The pressure thus exerted produced neither paralysis nor loss of consciousness and was exercised in such manner as to compress only the frontal lobes" (Stookey, 1963). I'm stunned how a word out of the mouth was cut in mid-syllable; I'm even more taken aback that Aubertin thought to use a kitchen utensil the way he did.

Auburtin wasn't attempting to show a difference between left and right brain function. He wielded his spatula to show that the front of the brain had to do with language, in defense of his father-in-law's pet theory. The father-in-law was a famous Parisian physician, Jean-Baptiste Bouillaud, who had been talking about the frontal lobes as parts of the brain dedicated to speech and language as early as 1825.

(If you're curious, Bouillaud's daughter's name was Elise. I haven't been able to learn much about her.)

The French school à la Brown-Séquard, Bouillaud, and Auburtin appealed to John. Functions like movement and speech could be demonstrated to be cortical at least in some way. By the late 1860's, two Germans, Gustave Fritsch and Eduard Hitzig, reproduced Luigi Rolando's experiments from over a half century before. Working in a garage, Fritsch and Hitzig electrically stimulated areas of cortex on one side of the brain's lateral surface in dogs–they used faradic current, which induces tetany if applied to muscle directly. Fritsch and Hitzig applied current to cortex here and there, then hindlimb, forelimb, or the face would move on the opposite side of dogs' bodies. The garage experiments wouldn't pass a research institutional review board today (the protocol's barbaric; the garage venue . . . just inappropriate), but the findings supported John's observations about a relationship between cerebral cortex and the movement of body parts.

What about John and the theory of evolution?

*

"To evolve," from Latin, is "to unroll." Highly evolved activities, like human speech or coordinated movements like dancing or just walking on two legs, don't happen in the manner of a *deus ex machina*. John wondered whether a seizure rolled back the clock of brain development. Actually, in any brain disease, could we retreat in evolutionary time–or: as John wrote himself, could cortical function "undevelop" (Jackson, 1884)?

Here's a story to explain more about going backwards.

One of John's patients was a government clerk (Jackson, 1866). The clerk had been well educated in British schools. From 1863 to 1865, he had four partial seizures, all involving the left side of his body. Early in 1865, more seizures, again partial, involved his right, not the left body. There was a problem with his speech after the right-body seizures. He was "incoherent." But his incoherent speech didn't last for long.

Some weeks later, John met the clerk again, by happenstance, on a London street. The clerk seemed healthy, not weak on either side of his body. He spoke fluently in a long conversation during which, John wrote, "if he had made the slightest mistake of any sort, I should have caught it at once." But the clerk seemed just fine.

Then the patient volunteered his own sense of his problem, as John describes it: "On my remarking that I had not detected any defect of speech, the patient said that his speech was imperfect 'when anything came on him suddenly,' or when he was not thinking particularly of what he was saying. His greatest trouble, however, was in writing. He had no difficulty in penmanship; on the contrary, it was beautiful. His trouble was that he could not readily find the proper words, and those he wrote he often spelled incorrectly." In an effort "to write a tolerably correct letter," the clerk had a strategy. He wrote drafts.

Here's a sample first draft of a letter. The crossed-out words are the clerk's own self-corrections:

> I glad to say that I am going on all right, and I home [hope] to continue to do so. I galy [daily] take a long walk, and do not find the configue [fatigue] as I formerly did. I am aglie agissue agligere to stop and think ~~what~~ how ~~spell~~ the wors [words] are spelt. I can ver ger generly go on verly well in may makeing the second copy.

Here's the second draft:

> I am glad to say that I am going on all right, and I hope to continue to do so. I daly take a long walk, and do not find the fatigue as I formerly did. I am oblige to stop and think as to how as to how the words are spell. I can generaly go on ~~verly~~ very well in making the second copy.

Transcribing a passage from a magazine (London's *Saturday Review*) was difficult for the clerk. Here's the original text, which John read aloud to him:

> The man whose mind is entirely taken up with small details, fancies he has a right to sneer at every one gifted with less minute knowledge. Because he can grease the wheels and tighten the screws of machinery he fancies himself an authority on the laws of motion.

Here's the clerk's transcription:

> The mand woos minds is entirely taken out with sall detales, sances he has a right to seen at every one fisted with lest minute nowledge. Begase Begause he gan crease the weels and bighten the schrees of masheenery he sances himself an authority on the laus of mosien.

What can we infer about the clerk's problem? Maybe in his "undevelopment" we learn about how we first develop the ability to express ourselves.

Looking at the clerk's transcription from the *Saturday Review*, letters and words seem put together as a child would do ("weels" for "wheels"). Sometimes, there's a drop-out of sense (I don't understand "bighten the schrees," for example).

I somewhat understand "schrees of masheenery," because I recognize "masheenery;" but I don't understand "The mand woos minds . . . with sall detales . . . "

With the actual passage in front of us, meaning gets clearer in the clerk's version. But, without the original, we have a garbled message. We have to ask, "Say again?" or "Write that again." And writing repeated drafts was the clerk's strategy.

Think about where we've been in our own personal development, since the time of pre-school: consider all the trial and error involved. Once upon a time, a child converted sounds to letters. Then she or he combined letters, then words, and somehow, eventually, linked words back to sounds. Especially in the clerk's transcript from the *Saturday Review*, I think we witness him going back to phonemes and phonetics, as if he had become an early grade-schooler again. He retreats as he tries to move forward.

*

When we think about a cortical process, maybe we shouldn't obsess too much over "schrees" of the "masheenery." Even if you know about parts of the brain (for example, the left versus the right cerebral hemisphere), it doesn't mean that you understand the laws that make for normal cortical function. Those laws have evolved in time, and time can go backwards in brain disease. That's what John Hughlings Jackson believed.

3.

Paris, 1861-1865

Xaxier Bichat moved to Paris from southeastern Lyon in post-revolutionary France, in 1793 or 1794. Anatomy was his life. He slept in morgues "to be able to dissect cadavers by day" (Shoja et al., 2008). Perhaps infamously, he wrote that "Two parts essentially alike in their structure cannot be different in their mode of acting" (quoted in Harris, 1999). More than sixty years later, Pierre-Paul Broca referred to Bichat's "law" of symmetry with respect to the brain:

> It is well known that the two hemispheres of the brain are perfectly similar; if the cerebral convolutions present slight and incidental variation from person to person, there are none that are appreciable from one side . . . to the other. Now there is one physiologic law, which everywhere else [in the body] is without exception, namely, that two organs that are equal and symmetrical have the same attributes, and it would be quite strange that this law should present here a marked exception (quoted in Berker et al., 1986).

Why shouldn't paired structures, like the two cerebral hemispheres, have like functions? Our two kidneys serve the same function physiologically, so why not the hemispheres of the brain?

Pierre-Paul Broca wasn't a neurologist or a neuroanatomist. He was a cigar-smoking general surgeon with polymathic interests, from painting, music, and rich food to the relationship between intelligence and brain size in so-called savages compared to modern Europeans. He helped to establish the Paris Anthropological Society in 1859. In the Spring of 1861, he was 36 years old.

On April 4, 1861 at the Paris Anthropological Society, Broca listened to the case reported by Jean-Baptiste Bouillaud's son-in-law, Ernest Aubertin, whom we mentioned in the last chapter.

On April 12, eight days later, someone asked Broca to see a patient named Leborgne for the surgical treatment of gangrene. There was nothing Broca could do for Leborgne, who died the following Wednesday, which was April 17.

On April 18, back at the Anthropological Society, Broca reported Leborgne's story, which only partly had to do with a speech problem (Broca, 1861a).

Leborgne's illness had progressed over decades. He suffered seizures as a younger man (we don't have details about the seizures), but he was able to hold a job as a hat maker for a while.

At age 30, Leborgne lost his speech. We don't know whether he lost it quickly or slowly. Two or three months later, Leborgne was admitted to the Bicêtre, an institution south of central Paris that was (then) part prison, part insane asylum, and, more or less, a hospital. You can visit *L'hôpital Bicêtre* today.

Bicêtre caregivers called him "Tan." Broca writes, "He understood all that was said to him . . . but, regardless of the question addressed to him, he always responded: *tan, tan*, with greatly varied gestures by means of which he succeeded in expressing most of his ideas [as well as an occasional explicative]." Broca added this about Tan's behavior, as described by ward attendants:

> Tan was regarded as being egotistical, vindictive, bad, and his comrades, who detested him, accused him even of being a thief . . . though this patient was at Bicêtre, one never thought of moving him to the division for the insane. He was considered, on the contrary, as a man perfectly responsible for his acts.

Had Leborgne always been detestable? Broca didn't think so.

After ten years at Bicêtre, Tan's right arm became completely paralyzed, afterwards his right leg as well, leaving him bedbound for six or seven years. His vision got worse. Also: "those who were close to him noted that his intelligence deteriorated a great deal in the final years."

The gangrene was nasty. It involved his right leg from foot to buttock.

Broca invited Ernest Auburtin (the one with the spatula) to examine Tan. Auburtin thought the problem to account for loss of speech must be towards the front of the brain—not a surprise, coming from Auburtin.

In 1865, after four years of collecting more cases like Tan's—and after what Broca called a lot of "pondering" over his experience—he localized a "site of the faculty of articulated speech" not just in the front brain, but to a specific place in the left frontal brain. He did so with a nod to Xavier Bichat (in the following passage, "encephalon," from Greek, means "marrow in the head" or the brain):

> In summary, the two halves of the encephalon, being perfectly identical from an anatomical point of view, cannot have different functions, but the more precocious

development of the left hemisphere makes us prone, in our first groping ways, to execute with that half of the brain the manual and intellectual actions that are most complex. Among such actions, one must certainly include the expression of ideas by means of language and, more particularly, articulate speech.

The two cortical hemispheres might not be identical from a developmental point of view, even if the anatomy looks symmetrical.

Across human cultures, there are more right handers than left handers. If a hemisphere can be dominant (as we say nowadays) for handedness, Broca thought it possible that a specific place in one hemisphere could be dominant for a human activity like language.

*

Broca retrieved Tan's brain after death. He didn't cut it up, but he studied it nevertheless. It weighed 987 grams, which is less than a typical normal weight, about 1,500 grams. Overlying the lateral left hemisphere, a cyst pressed from the outside. Broca punctured the cyst, and clear fluid drained out, to reveal a cavity the size of a chicken egg. Around the hole, some of the left brain's cortex felt soft, as if rotted.

Broca wondered about an analogy: what if the lack of articulate speech (like Tan's way of communicating, which wasn't fluent, despite cuss words) was like the state of a young child,

> ... a young child who already understands the language of those around him, who is sensitive to blame and praise, who points out with his fingers all the objects that he can name, who has acquired a crowd of simple

ideas, and who, to express these, can do nor more than stammer out a single syllable? (Broca, 1861b)

Tan's brain had "undeveloped," to use Hughlings Jackson's term. It undeveloped such that verbal output wasn't great, but maybe he understood a lot. Somehow he occasionally got his wishes across to his attendants, who (Tan realized) didn't like him very much.

Tan's brain is still around. People have MRI'd it (Dronkers et al., 2007). The brain sat in a jar of fixative for about 150 years, so conclusions are tentative. But the entire left hemisphere, including its white matter, doesn't look so good, and we're not just talking about the cortical hole towards the front on the left side. The right hemisphere isn't perfect either, especially in its white matter. The authors of the 2007 study talk about how the MR findings are "far deeper" than Broca was able to report.

"Deep" refers to a white matter issue, deep to cortex.

4.

Breslau and Vienna, 1874

Karl (or Carl) Wernicke, all of 26 years old in 1874, published "The Aphasia Symptom Complex: A Psychological Study on an Anatomical Basis" in what is now Poland's city of Wroclaw. Back then, the city was called Breslau, a major industrial center of Silesia and Prussia throughout the late 19th century.

His little book, only about 70 pages long, was brash. Wernicke knew about Broca. Wernicke's admiration for the surgeon was matched only by his disbelief that speech localized just to the front part of the brain.

Here I'll quote Wernicke, borrowing the way old German books once emphasized important sentences, with spaces between every important letter: "T h e   e n t i r e   s u r f a c e   o f   t h e   b r a i n   c a n   b e   d i v i d e d   i n t o   t w o   l a r g e   a r e a s   o f   f u n c t i o n a l l y   d i f f e r e n t   s i g n i f i c a n c e . . ." (Wernicke, 1874). The two large areas are: a frontal part (in front of the central sulcus of Rolando and above the Sylvian fissure) and, on the other hand, just about everywhere else in the cerebral cortex.

Wernicke said that the frontal brain had to do with movement–all kinds of movements, including speech. The second large area (the rest of the cortex) was sensory, containing what he called "memory images" of past sensory impressions. Frontal brain and other brain parts are connected. Wernicke's book is all about white-matter connections deep to cortex.

*

When I read Wernicke's book, it helps me to think about how listening influences how we speak. Think about an experiment that psychologists have performed many times: listen to your own voice through headphones as you speak, but, in the experiment, what you hear is delayed by a fraction of a second. Gobs of errors start to happen. You might mispronounce words, omit words (if you are reading out loud from a book), substitute words, or leave off word endings. How, when, and what we hear influences how we speak (Yates, 1963 and Hickock et al., 2011).

In Wernicke's opinion, language—including reading, speaking, hearing, and whatever else constitutes a language—wasn't an issue of a single location. He thought about white matter connecting the front part of the brain with other parts of the brain. "I have succeeded, by means of fiber dissections," he says (although others, like J. C. Reil and Karl Burdach, had described such connections before he did), "in showing a characteristic arrangement of bundles of fibers which lie just under the cortex . . ." in the immediate area of the Sylvian fissure.

Now, about memory: for Wernicke, "memory images" are everywhere in the cortex. The nervous system, he said later in his career (in 1900), remembers by its very nature. Memory is "a special feature of the nervous system characterized by permanent modifications of nerve tissues as the result of stimulation" (quoted in Eggers, 1997). Memories have to link up somehow, and if they do, we have intact "psychic" or cortical function. If they don't we have psychic or cortical symptoms. "[P]sychic symptoms," he wrote in 1874, "may be caused by disruption of the connecting fibers involved in the association of psychic elements . . . All higher psychic functions likely implicate the cerebral white matter."

⁂

For the record, Wernicke says on the first page that he's indebted to Theodor Meynert for his ideas. Meynert, who, it's been said, possessed a "massive head surmounting a short body" like a bobble-head doll, had a gigantic reputation (Papez, 1953). A young Sigmund Freud described him as the single most brilliant man he had ever met. We have to learn more about Meynert so that we can understand Wernicke better. Meynert worked in Vienna.

So, we'll travel south of Breslau to the Austro-Hungarian empire. Wernicke spent six months in Vienna, capital of the empire, at some point between 1871 and the publication of his book.

*

Of the 7,526 students enrolled at the University of Vienna in 1874, about 1,000 attended medical school, according to an eye-witness report that year in *The British Medical Journal*. At that time, it seems students actually wanted to attend class (streaming video occurred later in history, as we know). At least five days a week, someone named Brücke, a physiologist, lectured in a room too small for his crowd of 885 medical students, so one needed a ticket to enter.

A 70-ish year-old man with Victorian muttonchops, named Rokitansky, ran the school. Meynert, with his massive head, held courses about the brain that were "unrivaled . . . probably unique in Europe," according to the British visitor (Anonymous, 1874). There were other big names in Vienna. Billroth, a surgeon, worked at the nearby Vienna General Hospital, removing whole stomachs to treat gastric cancer; he taught 509 students besides.

Rokitansky with the muttonchops prided himself that the University of Vienna taught histology, then a relatively new discipline in German-speaking schools. Histology, from the Greek, is the study of *histos*, which is a web, mast, or a beam–that is, histology is the study of microscopically small webs, masts, and beams.

Theodor Meynert learned two important things histologically.

First, not all cerebral cortex looks the same. He hand-sliced cortex with a razor, fixed his material in alcohol, and stained it with either carmine or gold (Seitelberger, 1997). When he compared slices of cortex from different areas, he saw differences in layers of cortical cells. His brain slices were crude.

Later, in Berlin, Korbinian Brodmann identified 44 cortical areas, differentiated by layering discerned by microscope, in papers published from 1903 to 1909. (There's controversy over the final tally of all Brodmann's areas–some say there are 52; some say areas 13-16 and 48-51 don't exist [Olry and Haines, 2010].) In Vienna, Constantin von Economo described 109 areas in 1929. Back in Germany, the husband-and-wife team of Cécile and Oskar Vogt had the number as high as the 200's in 1919. Some people complain that looking microscopically for sharp boundaries in cortex can be taken "to absurd lengths" (Carpenter and Sutin, 1983).

Sure. A lot of education is absurd. But I have a question: if grey matter isn't all the same, can the same be said of white matter?

Here is Meynert's second observation at his microscope: subcortical white matter tracts are of different types, too. Fiber destinations distinguished the types. There are fibers that project to places like the spinal cord . . . or, fibers that connect the two hemispheres from left to right and vice versa . . . or, fibers that connect cortical areas within a single hemisphere. At very least, there are three types. Meynert wrote about cortex and white matter as if describing the whole earth as a nervous network, with "colonies of living beings, capable of consciousness, connected with each other with feeling threads and grasping tentacles, and controlling their image of the world." Wernicke also noticed fibers, especially what he called a spider's web, full of filaments, in the area of Sylvian fissure.

*

Getting back to Wernicke and language: he describes a second kind of speech disturbance, second only to Broca's descriptions. If you read Wernicke's cases (ten of them), you'd find it odd that a language problem associated with focally damaged cortex can't quite be found (Mathews et al., 1994). Maybe his first case is the purest example of what he wants to describe. But she got better before anyone could look at her brain.

Her name was Suzanne Adam. She was fifty-nine years old, a widow with one son. She looked frail. On March 1, 1874, she became abruptly dizzy and she had a headache. She went to bed in the afternoon; she traveled to hospital the following day. When some admitting doctors examined her, they commented about how confused she sounded. She could describe her headache and dizziness, but every once in awhile she'd use a nonsense word or a phrase that the doctors didn't understand. She could make perfect sense, but she didn't always. Wernicke himself examined her on March 7 at the earliest, in any event some days after the start of her problem.

She responded "yes" to the sound of her own name, but also to any other name.

When first asked to name some objects presented to her, including a hat, pencil, clock, and handkerchief, she did so correctly, but on retesting she had no idea how to answer.

On daily rounds that followed, she might correctly show her tongue when asked by a doctor, but if asked to do something else ("take the glass from the chair"), she'd show her tongue, close her eyes, or show her teeth. Evidently, she watched how rounds were conducted from bed to bed in the open ward; she mimicked how others showed their tongues to the doctor.

She could recite 14 lines of a prayer without error.

When presented a pencil, she took it in her hand correctly, put nib to paper, but produced only scribbles and single strokes.

By March 15 (two weeks after the attack of dizziness and headache), she improved. She responded to her own name, not to unfamiliar ones. On March 18, Wernicke records the following exchange between himself and Suzanne:

Dr. W:	Do you need anything?
Ms. Adam:	Oh my, now who would anyone say something to me . . . [with a friendly demeanor] . . . But I still do not know . . . to whom I should say someone.
Dr. W:	Is this a pencil?
Ms. Adam:	I do not know now what it is called. I recognize it very well. I have already swelled middle [that's my translation, your guess is as good as mine] with it . . . I know very well how it really comes to be called. I cannot remember it.

Next, she identified a clock (a clock on the wall, I think), sort of:

> Ms. Adam: A watch (speaking quietly) . . . a pocket… (speaking more loudly)… a pocket watch . . . a very fine one.

As said, there's no brain to study in Ms. Adam's case. After she got better, I guess she went home.

Wernicke does provide details about brains at autopsy in four of his ten patients. The cortical problem in those brains couldn't be called precise. In three cases, the temporal lobe in the left brain was involved in a big way–basically, there was damage more behind the central sulcus than in front of it. The fourth case involved an impressive abscess that occupied most of the left temporal lobe.

*

To find a more exquisite single case, we should head back to Vienna, to a basement library of the Billroth House of the Viennese Society of Physicians.

In 1992, someone happened upon a mis-shelved volume of the *Medical Yearbook of the House of the Imperial and Royal Society of Physicians in Vienna* from 1866. In that particular volume, there's a case report by Theodor Meynert (Whitaker and Etlinger, 1993). Wernicke doesn't mention any such paper in his book.

Here's a summary of Meynert's case report.

A 23-year old woman had a known history of heart disease. About two weeks before she died for reasons that aren't made clear, she experienced, in Meynert's words, "a sudden inhibition of expressive speech" without weakness on either side of her body. Her words came out strangely: a "hand" was a "yellow," for example. It wasn't a yellow hand, just a "yellow."

At autopsy, she had just one small area where cortex had infarcted, in the left brain, in the temporal lobe, in the area of the Sylvian fissure, not towards the front of the brain but, instead, far behind the central sulcus. The rest of the brain was fine, but maybe the white matter underneath the cortex didn't look so good. The report didn't say exactly.

*

After 1874, one really can't talk about brain function without thinking about grey and white matter together.

5.

Leipzig, 1898

Paul Emil Flechsig of Leipzig, Germany seems upset. Here he is in 1901, annoyed at someone who didn't use the correct Flechsigian brain diagrams, which Flechsig published in 1898:

> . . . useless. They are neither copies of my drawings of 1898 . . . nor of any other illustrations whatever that have been published by me. They are simply of the nature of misconceptions . . . incomplete . . . [they] can only lead to confusion (Flechsig, 1901).

What was so important about his own drawings? For one thing, they have to do with white matter in relation to the cortex.

Flechsig studied full-term infant brains pathologically; we don't how or why the babies died. He noticed that some, not all, of the white matter beneath the cortex was visible to the naked eye. If white matter is visible to the naked eye, it doesn't mean that it has become fully mature–whatever "full" "maturity" might be.

We expect human brains to get more complex in post-natal development, because babies do less than adults. Newborns don't talk in full sentences and they don't tell lies. But what's the significance of areas "invested with medullary substance [white matter]"? Of note, large areas of the cortical surface *aren't* invested with white matter/medullary substance at birth.

Let Flechsig speak for himself: "primordial zones" invested with medullary substance contain "the points of entrance of all the channels conveying sensory impressions to the cortex . . . The individual sensory areas are separated from one another by wide tracts of cortex . . . in which sensory fibers cannot be followed up."

*

Let's think about his observation for a moment. We learn about the world through the five basic senses:

HEARING
SIGHT
SMELL
TASTE
TOUCH

Are they separate? If they are, how do we hold something, look at it, sniff it, bite into it, and even listen to it, to decide that–say–it's a crisp apple? It makes some sense that you don't exactly taste what you hear–so maybe those two senses could be called separate. But I like crisp apples, not soft ones–they sound and taste better to me. You might have a different preference in apples.

According to Flechsig, the brain in humans has particular points of entry into that brain for hearing, sight, and so on, like five people entering a building through different doors. The five people never exactly meet; they never shake hands (in terms of "person-to-person," direct axonal connections). If those people had names, they might be:

>   CRISP
>   RED
>   FRESH
>   SWEET
>   FIRM

Newborns don't bite into crisp apples, so what am I talking about? Hang on. What about this set of people?

>   COO
>   BROWN EYES
>   FLOWERY
>   MILKY
>   SOFT

How do you get from those names or sensations to an idea of "mother"? An idea of mom has to be put together somehow, probably not randomly.

*

For years, Paul Emil Flechsig lived in a cottage behind his clinic on the grounds of the University of Leipzig. When he retired, he said he owned the cottage, and he refused to leave. The university evicted him.

*

At very least, portions of the human cortex invested with white matter at birth have to do with our five senses. With that knowledge alone, we're in a position to brood—not skim—over very professorial material like this:

> In accordance with the principle of Flechsig (which is applicable to man and the other primates but not to subprimate forms), the primary projection areas now send their connexions primarily to the immediately adjacent association cortex (parakoniocortex); the long connections (either within a hemisphere or between hemispheres) between different cortical regions take place predominantly between parts of the association cortex (Geschwind, 1974).

I'll end our historical excursion over the last three chapters now. My next job is systematically to unpack the above passage by Norman Geschwind, who died in 1984 in his office (so legend attests) at the too-young age of 58.

I'll need the next two chapters to do my work. By the way, his reference to Flechsig is the tip of a proverbial iceberg, because we'll need to revisit Jacksonian undevelopment, Broca's hardly original interest in the frontal brain (Bouillaud and Aubertin entertained the idea well before he did), Wernicke and his Meynert-inspired interest in subcortical connections, and the irascible, evicted Flechsig just to understand the implications of Geschwind's single, very dense, professorial sentence.

6.

Sound

Let's start with the sound of the apple.

Over years of teaching, I've given the auditory pathway embarrassingly short shrift. Right now is an opportunity to make some amends.

Since communication by sound antedates written text of any kind in history, a discussion of language should attend, carefully, to hearing.

There's a more personal motivation, separate from my prep for this short book. In recent years, I've tried to pick up new languages, just to be able to converse a bit in foreign places where I get invited to teach. Listening to a strange language is interesting neurologically. It's been observed that a problem in understanding foreign speech is, in no small part, a problem in actually hearing speech. A.R. Luria explains that a person who doesn't know a foreign language not only does not understand it, but also, in effect, she or he doesn't *hear* it–i.e., does not "systematize the sounds of speech." Instead, what's heard is just a stream, endlessly meaningless it often seems, of sounds (Luria, 1980).

Can that person "hear"?

*

Transduction of sound in air to action potentials happens at the hair cell, the specialized mechanoreceptor involved both in the cochlear and vestibular functions of cranial nerve VIII. If you're in search of a simple analogy to understand the cochlea, you'd profit from Nolte (1999), who himself borrowed from a 1975 textbook.

Imagine a cylinder open on both ends. The open ends are covered by pliant membranes–on the top, an "oval window," on top of which the stapes sits; on the bottom, a "round window."

In the middle of the cylinder there's a third membrane, also pliant. This middle membrane has an opening on one end, where the membrane would otherwise attach to the inside of the cylinder. That hole we'll call the helicotrema, which is a conduit between upper and lower halves of the cylinder's interior. Both the upper and lower halves are filled with one type of lymphatic fluid.

Populate the middle membrane with hair cells along its entire length.

Next comes the interesting, if surreal part of the exercise: imagine a dramatic elongation of the cylinder along its horizontal axis, with the helicotrema at the apex of the elongation. The basic compartments are all present as you elongate: upper half (scala vestibuli, contiguous with the vestibular apparatus), lower half (scala tympani, which is in contact with the "second" tympanic membrane–i.e., the round window), and our middle membrane. Coil up what you've created; you've constructed an elementary cochlea, which now resembles a snail's shell.

An apple crunch, at 60 or so crisp decibels, causes stapes to push and pull at the oval window. Both the middle membrane and round window will also move, because lymphatic fluid in the cylinder (so-called perilymph, similar in composition to sodium-rich cerebrospinal fluid) moves in response to action at the oval window. Push at the oval window; there will be initial downward displacement of the middle membrane, and a bulge outward at the round window. Perilymph circulates from the cylinder's upper half to its lower half via the helicotrema. With more pushing and pulling at the oval window, the middle membrane deforms as if a wave runs through it.

"Middle membrane," which we have populated with hair cells, is a simplification. It refers collectively to all the structures and contents of the scala media, or membranous labyrinth, including outer and inner hair cells in the Organ of Corti. The scala media, in fact, is a third compartment in our model, different from the scalae vestibuli and tympani. It's filled with endolymph rather than perilymph. Endolymph is potassium rich, like the chemical composition *inside* cells of the body.

There's sanity to the simplification, however: when we think of the scala media as a single, long middle membrane, we begin to understand tonotopic or cochleotopic organization. Hair cell transduction and cochlear nerve transmission that result from sounds at particular frequencies depend on the location of hair cells on the (elongated) middle membrane.

*

Sensory afferents to the brain have ganglia; in the case of the cochlear division of cranial nerve VIII, it's the spiral ganglion, the location of cell bodies of primary auditory afferents. Cochlear fibers of cranial nerve VIII–let's discuss the left one–enter the brainstem at the left pontomedullary junction; they head to one of two left cochlear nuclei (one dorsal, one ventral) which drape like a puddled curtain over the lateral edge of the left inferior cerebellar peduncle. Second-order neurons arise from the left cochlear nuclei. Their axons head to the left superior olivary nucleus, which sits atop the upper/rostral end of the left facial nucleus in the pons.

Nature is always more complicated than what we teach. The first step in the auditory pathway, from cochlear nuclei to superior olivary nucleus, is a case in point. I'll dwell on some minutiae, but they should interest us:

1. There are two cochlear nuclei. Second-order axons arising from dorsal nucleus seem to take a very different route to rostral points than those arising from the ventral nucleus.

2. The superior olivary nucleus (sometimes divided into two nuclei, one medial and one lateral) receives fibers from *ventral* cochlear nucleus as part of a "binaural sound localization stream."

3. Some fibers arising from *dorsal* cochlear nucleus simply ascend as second-order axons towards rostral brainstem (we'll comment to where in a moment). Why is there a second "stream" which presumably differs from one having to do with "binaural sound localization"?

On many occasions, I've said that the superior olivary nucleus, a destination of second-order neurons, is *the* first place in the central nervous system where there's bilateral representation of sound. A central lesion, I've taught, can result in strictly unilateral hearing loss if the lesion is "infranuclear"—i.e., caudal to the superior olivary nucleus—as if the lesion were in cranial nerve VIII itself. Considering the subject in greater detail, I feel both justified and stupid.

Left superior olivary nucleus receives second-order neurons from both the left (ipsilateral) and right (contralateral) cochlear nuclei. Right fibers get to the left side via the trapezoid body, a white-matter tract that passes transversely in the axial plane; it can be found roughly at the level of the cranial nerve VI nuclei in the pons. Some, not all, contralateral fibers (those that have arisen from right cochlear nucleus) synapse in the left superior olivary nucleus. If a synapse does occur in left superior olivary nucleus, a third-order axon passes into left lateral lemniscus, heading to left inferior colliculus.

Some second-order axons arising from left cochlear nuclei never cross the midline, and will ascend to more rostral destinations ipsilaterally with or without synapsing in left superior olivary nucleus. In other words, there's a partial, not complete decussation of left cochlear nuclear fibers—a situation akin to the optic chiasm (the partial decussation happens at the superior olivary nucleus).

Now we revisit the curiosity of the dorsal cochlear nucleus. Second-order fibers arising from it often (not always) pass without decussation into the ipsilateral lateral lemniscus.

So, left dorsal-cochlear, second-order neurons travel along with second-or third-order neurons from contralateral and ipsilateral cochlear nuclei, via lateral lemniscus, towards inferior colliculus . . . to accomplish what?

Here's where I discover my stupidity (not too strong a word). If I'm quite deaf in one ear, don't I still appreciate when there's a sound, for example, above my head?

Binaural processing happens at multiple levels at and rostral to the superior olivary nucleus, because of cross connections like the trapezoid body and others—e.g., the commissure of Probst, which is another transverse conduit like the trapezoid body (Probst's commissure connects lateral lemnisci from side to side) or, more superiorly, the commissure of the inferior colliculi.

The "stream" arising from left dorsal cochlear nucleus ends, mainly, in inferior colliculus. At the inferior colliculus, inputs from many places converge to process sound localization in the vertical plane, among other "complex" aspects of sound (Pickles, 2015).

The last paragraph invites a question or two. As a meaningless sound, a crunch of fruit or a snap above one's head has frequencies that map tonotopically at the cochlea. But to listen, really listen, involves other aspects: where the sound is; how long it lasts; who's making the sound; and what it sounds *like*. Isn't it foolish to think that the requisite and prerequisite processing of data happens only after one anatomical site? Could processing start as early as the division between dorsal and ventral cochlear nuclei or even earlier, at the Organ of Corti?

7.

Arrival at Primary Auditory Cortex

We've alluded to these structures of the brainstem: cochlear nuclei (dorsal and ventral), superior olivary nuclei, the trapezoid body, lateral lemnisci and their commissure, and the inferior colliculi and their commissure.

I've not mentioned nuclei of the trapezoid body, ventral and dorsal nuclei of the lateral lemniscus, or much of anything substantive about the inferior colliculi. But it's a safe surmise that each of these stations (which crosstalk to each other, across the brainstem's midline) probably processes cochlear input in some way—the information could relate to pitch, tone, volume, timing, location, background vs. foreground noise, or what have you.

It seems a short couple of steps from inferior colliculus in midbrain, via medial geniculate nucleus (or body) of thalamus, to primary auditory cortex. The primary auditory cortex is a "primary projection area" in Geschwind's parlance and a "primordial zone" in Flechsig's nomenclature. There's yet another name for primary auditory cortex which more usefully locates where the thing is in the brain: Heschl's transverse temporal gyrus (some refer to gyri), a portion of the temporal, not frontal, lobe. To find it, you have to look inside the Sylvian fissure at the temporal lobe's superior, otherwise hidden surface. (Anatomist Richard Ladislaus Heschl worked at the University of Vienna early and late in his career in the 19th century. Rokitansky with his muttonchops was Heschl's early mentor.)

In light of what we've said about the likelihood of processing at each station (not relay station) in the auditory pathway, it should come as no surprise that the final connection ending in cortex, from medial geniculate nucleus, simply is not trivial.

Nor have I forgotten my task from chapter five, namely, to explain Geschwind's thoughts about cortical organization when it comes to a primary sensory modality. But long before we arrive at temporal-lobe cortex, as we trace just one pathway heading there, we really discuss the development of a perception. As we know from John Hughlings Jackson, where there's development, there can be undevelopment when things go wrong.

*

What is a (primary) sensory cortex? Can it be characterized histologically? The answer—of course there's an answer, because why else would a teacher ask those particular questions?—has to do with appearance of dust.

We're not talking about heaps of dust in a long-neglected place. If I look at my desktop in the morning, with sunlight oblique to the surface, I see a patina of new dust. It's uniform like an evanescently thin sheet of punctate grey. In a desk drawer, I have a cloth and some dust spray. I dust. I'm tidy, but I wipe away the appearance, speaking histologically, of koniocortex (*konios*, Greek, for dust). Dust on my desktop doesn't organize into six neocortical layers. But to my eye looking at koniocortex, laminations aren't immediately apparent either;

I see an expanse of very small neurons like so many particles of dust on my morning desk.

The take-home is: there's histological monotony to the appearance of primary sensory cortices.

I read (Kaas et al., 1999b) that the so-called "core" of primary auditory cortex is koniocellular, but a "belt," which surrounds the core, is not. Around the "belt" is a "parabelt," which also is not koniocellular. Perhaps I finally understand what Geschwind means by "parakoniocortex." Let me cut and paste the relevant passage for you: "the primary projection areas now send their connexions primarily to the immediately adjacent association cortex (parakoniocortex)." He refers to what later researchers describe as a "belt," which wraps around a "core," or perhaps to "parabelt" which is outside the belt.

The core is tripartite.

Wait. Is the (primary) auditory cortex just one place or more than one place?

Enigmatic answer: Yes.

*

Students dislike such answers, I know. But it's no less sketchy to say that there are three cores. "The" core responds to tones.

Step back, or upstream, to the medial geniculate nucleus, which has three divisions distinguished (in part) by the areas to which they respectively connect. Projections from *ventral* medial geniculate nucleus input to the core. The belt receives projections from no less than four places: the core, the *dorsal* and *medial* divisions of medial geniculate nucleus, and, only to a much lesser degree, from ventral medial geniculate nucleus. Parabelt receives input mainly from belt, but also from dorsal and medial divisions of medial geniculate nucleus and from other thalamic subnuclei and nuclei, including pulvinar. The major difference between ventral, dorsal, and medial divisions of medial geniculate nucleus is tonotopic or cochleotopic organization. Only the ventral division has it.

Roughly 25 years ago, the core *was* the classical primary auditory cortex (abbreviated A1). Since then we've learned that there are three cochleotopic maps in the core–A1 being one of them. So anatomists today refer to three core fields, all of which are koniocellular, and all of which receive axons exclusively from the tonotopically organized ventral division of medial geniculate nucleus. A single core neuron in any of the three cochlear maps of the core responds to "a" characteristic frequency with some wiggle room, about one-third of an octave. By contrast, in the rostral parabelt (located on the lateral brain surface, not buried inside the Sylvian fissure; parabelt is part of the superior temporal gyrus), neurons there response to white noise rather than tones.

What is the whiteness of noise? I suppose like white light it has many components that comprise it–we start with tones only, then we construct "noise."

At this moment, I recall the clerk from chapter two trying to correspond in a letter (in his first draft): "I can ver ger generly go on verly well . . ." His effort isn't noise, not just tones either; possibly, it's something beyond noise, because it has something akin to meaning.

*

If I've done my job as a teacher, the reader's still with me; if not, this book is already in a bin somewhere.

It's time to unpack–or, rather, interpret and rewrite–Geschwind from 1974:

"*In accordance with the principle of Flechsig (which is applicable to man and the other primates but not to subprimate forms)* . . ." Paul

Emil Flechsig of Leipzig happened upon a kind of revelation especially pertinent to humans and primates. His "principle" is *not* . . .

". . . *the primary projection areas now send their connexions primarily to the immediately adjacent association cortex (parakoniocortex)*. . . " . . . to repeat, is *not* that primary projection areas of cortex, like primary auditory cortex, project to immediately adjacent areas. Neurons have axons that connect to many places. Why wouldn't there be connections ("connexions") to nearest-neighbor cortex? Theodor Meynert observed as much at his microscope in Vienna. Flechsig's principle is that primary sensory areas don't communicate directly with each other in primates and humans.

". . . *the long connexions (either within a hemisphere or between hemispheres) between different cortical regions take place predominantly between parts of the association cortex.*" Connectivity, like myelination, isn't unique to primates and humans. When Wernicke divided the whole brain into frontal/motor and, well, everything else/sensory (non-frontal brain occupies itself with sensation *a lot*: think about all the cortical space dedicated just to visual and auditory processing), he thought that connections were so important that all higher functions had to implicate white matter.

From a different point of view, what seems perfectly unique in the primate and human brain is the exaggerated cortical territory between (beyond) so-called unimodal association areas–e.g., unimodal belt and parabelt connections lead afield from the core, and very far afield from the parabelt, as far as the prefrontal brain (Kaas and Hackett, 1999a).

Beyond unimodal association areas, we have what Flechsig called "wide tracts of cortex . . . in which sensory fibers cannot be followed up," or what A.R. Luria (1966 and 1980) called tertiary zones (e.g., core = primary; belt/parabelt = secondary; beyond parabelt = tertiary), or what we currently describe as "multimodal" (or "heteromodal") association areas.

In a rewind of evolution, what do we lose in terms of anatomical parts if we undevelop a primate or human brain? I'd wonder about Luria's tertiary zones, about multimodality.

8.

Pierre Marie's Issue

Academics have their testy moments as other people do. Pierre Marie (1853-1940)–who established a neurological service at Bicêtre long after Tan's time there, who was an ardent student of Jean-Martin Charcot, and who eventually succeeded (in his 60's, though Marie lived well into his 80's) to Charcot's professorship at the Salpêtrière in eastern Paris–was a king of snark when it came to Broca's "area." I base my claim on the title of a paper from 1906: *"La Troisième Circonvolution Frontal Gauche ne Joue aucun Role Spéciale dans la Fonction du Langage* [The third left frontal convolution plays no special role whatsoever in the function of language]" (quoted in Finger, 1994). For our purposes, we can call the third frontal convolution, or pars opercularis of the inferior frontal gyrus, "Broca's area." But there's debate to this day over whether it has clear boundaries.

Another of Broca's critics, Wernicke, would be subject to similar criticism regarding localization of *his own* area, which we say is roughly in the posterior third of the superior temporal gyrus (in the left hemisphere for most of us). A modern heir to Wernicke writes, "Wernicke's area has no universally accepted boundary. It is usually defined as 'the region which causes Wernicke's aphasia when damaged'" (Mesulam, 2000). That's more funny than vicious, I think.

As a bedside clinician, part of me appreciates Marie's reduction of complexity to rules that are serviceable and, above all, simple. He wrote in the 1906 paper: "We have seen, as a matter of fact, that the only notable difference between the aphasia of Wernicke and the aphasia of Broca is that in the first, patients speak more or less badly, while in the second they do not speak at all. But in both forms, one finds that intellectual deficit which had as its immediate consequence difficulty in understanding sentences which are a little bit complicated and difficulty with or the total loss of reading and writing." According to Marie's "rule" for the bedside evaluation of language, we could say the following about cases that we've encountered so far in this monograph:

1. John's government clerk had a problem especially with writing. He exhibited, just as he described of himself, what modern aphasiologists call *la conduite d'approche* or "successive attempts to self-correct" (Bernal and Ardila, 2009). He understood language well enough to take dictation, though very imperfectly. Bedside conclusion: probably not a frontal aphasia.
2. Tan couldn't speak, but he seemed to understand at least something of his environment at Bicêtre, maybe especially how the attendants came to dislike him. (We didn't explore Broca's second clinical case, who was a man named Lelong with a very limited vocabulary—"*oui*," "*non*," "*toujours*," maybe another word or two in French. He essentially had no speech. He could not write.) Bedside conclusion in both cases: probably frontal. The hint is that they are both Broca's cases. But how focal is the lesion in either case? Perhaps not focal at all.
3. Regarding Suzanne Adam, I wonder: could she understand Wernicke? We don't know where the lesion(s) was/were. According to Marie's rule, however, the bedside conclusion

would be: probably not a frontal aphasia. Why? She speaks more or less badly, but she speaks.

4. In the case of Meynert's 23 year-old woman, a human hand was a "yellow" (not a yellow hand, just a "yellow"). Is the word "yellow" (*gelb* in German) all that different from the word "hand" (*hand* in German)? Both are four-letter words with one vowel; in both cases, there's one vowel tone with consonants surrounding it. Her words, Meynert said, "came out strangely"–which suggests to me that substitutions like *gelb* for *hand* happened in the context of fluent verbal output. Bedside conclusion: probably not a frontal aphasia.

Can one begin to understand why Marie's real issue wasn't so opprobrious as the title of his 1906 paper? Many aphasias look like cases 1, 3, and 4; fewer have features of case 2, except in the common instance of an aphasia, more global than focal, with a right hemiplegia and a right visual field cut–in such a case, one barely needs either a neurologist or a brain image to envision the global destruction of left hemisphere.

*

My intent is not to subtract from lovely analyses that aphasiologists perform today with fastidious care. Rather, I'm interested in the impression of a language problem. In our routine bedside examination, after we've simply listened for a while, we test naming, repetition, and comprehension; we obtain a sample of writing. We look at the penned words. Sometimes, we just want to see if pen meaningfully hits paper at all. We listen to language out of the mouth of patients, attentive to missteps for which we have studious names.

Today, let's admit, we're not far from Marie's pragmatism at the bedside, because we're interested to discover, at a glance if possible, where the nidus of a problem might be in what we now fancifully call a distributed language network.

(I'm fully aware that a more thorough examination of language explores, for example, the components of Gerstmann syndrome, or the features of alexia without agraphia, or clues to reveal any of a number of well-described entities in neurology. But perhaps a personally embarrassing story will help explain my approach in the remaining chapters.)

As a chief neurology resident in Boston a long time ago, naturally I wanted to be a fountain of knowledge and a paragon of acumen for junior residents and students. I recall teaching one day about *paraphrasic* errors in dysphasic speech–the word that came out of my mouth was "para-'phrasic.'" I thought I did a passable job describing phonemic or literal vs. semantic or verbal substitutions, etc. But "para-'phrasic'" kept coming out of my chief-residential mouth, until a junior resident, whose look of condescending disgust I recall to this moment, said "oh, for God's sake, the word is para*phasic*."

It's hard to retain dignity under such circumstances. One extra "r," and it seemed my future had already been cast in shadow. At least, I learned not to speak outside my ken. To this very day.

I'm neither an aphasiologist nor a network theorist, but I am fundamentally interested in language. I seek plain-spoken-ness like Pierre Marie, but without other tendentious "issues.")

One way to deconstruct–to begin to understand–a distributed network is to glean what multimodality means and how it operates. In the next two chapters, we'll look at two multimodal areas, one temporo-parietal-occipital and the other (more mysterious perhaps) frontal-prefrontal.

9.

A Problem With Naming, Part I

In front of me, I have *The Assessment of Aphasia and Related Disorders*, by Goodglass and Kaplan, in its second edition (1983), because it's the book I used in my training. It's remarkable to reflect how often over 30 years I've taught what the authors wrote, especially the first sentence of what follows, that "[n]aming to visual presentation is a universally used test for aphasia since virtually all aphasic patients have some loss of capacity to perform. While it may be described as a visual input/oral output task, there is reason to believe that this is a simplistic view that does not do justice to the intervening processes."

Naturally we're interested in the intervening processes. But my approach is not–I hope it's not–akin to contemporary articles that presume to tell us about "the neural basis" of object naming or some other aspect of human language. I'm interested to know more about just two things.

First, why is anomia or dysnomia so consistently characteristic of dominant hemispheric lesions? Second, in light of the fact that a hemisphere is a vast amount of neurological real estate, do problems with naming help us understand different locales of multimodal processing?

(Yes, I know I haven't yet discussed what multiple "modes" are involved. I ask for patience.)

*

The Boston Diagnostic Aphasia Examination is a Goodglass-Kaplan instrument with many sections. We'll refer only to portions of it for our discussion. For example, what's the difference between naming based on questions of this type–

What do we cut paper with?
or
What color is grass?

–as opposed to a battery of naming tests that explores seven different categories? The latter is a lengthier, more demanding test; here are the seven categories, with sample queries per category (patients are asked to identify objects, letters, etc. when the examiner points to a picture or image of the item to be named):

Objects:	"glove,"
	"feather"
Letters:	"R,"
	"L"
Geometric Forms:	"square,"
	"triangle"
Actions:	"sleeping,"
	"falling"
Numbers:	"1936,"
	"42"
Colors:	"blue,"

	"purple"
Body Parts:	"nose,"
	"shoulder"

Is a question such as "what do we cut paper with?" a test of naming or an interrogation about the verb "to cut"? Knives cut, as do scissors. The authors say: one seeks *response* (the name of an item) without a visual cue–that's nominally and exclusively what the test seeks to reveal. The lengthier test involves naming in multiple categories of objects after visual presentation of an item to be named. Both tests are scored not only on the basis of correct answers, but also on how long it takes for the answer to emerge after the requisite neural churning has been accomplished–or, in some cases, not accomplished.

To state the obvious, responsive naming ("what do we cut paper with?") is an aural test. Visual confrontation naming–the examiner points to an image–is both a visual and aural test, since the preliminary instructions need to be heard and understood, as is true as well for the responsive naming test. Results of the two tests in aphasic patients correlate with each other, in general. That is, a problem with responsive naming tends to be as severe as a problem in visual confrontation naming in aphasia. But there are exceptions. Let's consider two examples, one in this chapter and one in the next.

*

A 54 year-old man, whose previous work had to do with ship building, suffered an ischemic stroke. At first, his right body was affected both in terms of movement and sensation. He improved over three months to the point where he could move his right arm and hand rather well, but a "cortical sensory" deficit persisted in his right arm– and, it's reasonable to assume, also in his right hand.

I hope that the reader has had the experience of seeing and wondering about what happens in strokes with respect to the sense of touch, as opposed to what happens in polyneuropathies or polyradiculopathies. In a cortical deficit rather than a neuropathic one, it's not merely that you can't feel; there's a problem identifying abstract aspects of a sensation. With a pass of an examiner's finger on the skin, can the patient appreciate whether the movement is "up" vs. "down"? With palpation alone in the affected hand (with eyes closed), can that person identify what an object is? Place an American coin in that hand: can she or he appreciate the difference between a dime and a quarter, a quarter and a nickel? What if the coin were placed in the left, not the right hand?

I'd guess that the 54 year-old would have a problem both with the visual identification of any coin as well as with its tactile identification in either hand. I could be wrong. But we know from Goodglass and Kaplan that visual confrontation naming was poor across categories. His cumulative score, expressed as a percentile (100 being normal), was about 30. Why should his tactile naming be any different in either hand?

*

An anecdote.

A late teacher of mine once drew my attention to how aphasics explore sets of pictures with no instruction whatsoever about what to do in the test. He was curious about their eye movements–whether the eyes might reveal whether aphasics comprehended what's in view (Locke, 2014). The concept is interesting: to look around, *with* an anomia. What's that *like*? Maybe an aphasic person knows aspects of an object without an ability to name it. An anomia isn't necessarily either an agnosia or a failure to recognize–but in agnosia one can't name, because one doesn't recognize in the first place (Mesulam, 2000). In an anomia, one may not access the name, but yet . . . one could know the object of interest.

I wonder whether there isn't a relationship, in some cases, between dysnomia and (for lack of a better word) a hyper-nomia. If I look at grass, let's say I think of "the beautiful uncut hair of graves" (Walt Whitman in *Leaves of Grass*). How would the poetry score in the eyes of the examiner? Or, if I see "42," what if my response is "Jackie Robinson" or "Dodger" or (this next one is cryptic; you have to know about Bronx, not Brooklyn history) "cutter"? If the examiner interviewing me knew nothing of baseball, I might be admitted somewhere immediately.

*

What if we show the ship builder an American dime, or we place one in his hand, and we ask "is it a dime?" (The question differs from the visual-confrontation naming test, because in the latter an examiner never verbally identifies any item.) I wonder how he'd respond. I don't know, but, again, my guess is that he wouldn't do well.

Alternatively, let's say I'm wrong, as I often am. Maybe he readily acknowledges a penny as a cent, a dime as ten cents, etc. even if words "penny" and "dime" never come out of his mouth. Do we then say that he "knows" coins?

The interesting result is that he scored in the 90th percentile for responsive naming. Perhaps if he were asked "name the smallest American coin by size," he'd respond correctly. Or: was his relative success due to a knee-jerk reflexive quality in the answer "green" (for example) in response to "what color is grass?"

He comprehended verbal instructions, but he couldn't read or write. He couldn't spell words dictated to him. He often confused right from left. He was lousy at math (10th percentile).

What "modes" are involved, based on the clinical information provided? We're not told about a visual field defect or a cortical blindness—let's say there wasn't any such problem, for the sake of argument. Then why couldn't he identify objects presented visually? Responsive naming was almost normal, and he could understand verbal instructions, so why couldn't he take dictation? And, of course, we were told right off the bat about his cortical somatosensory problem on the right.

Lesion localization isn't the issue here; nor is the diagnosis attached to the 54 year-old's case (our textbook says, "anomic aphasia"—a term that has always struck me as redundant). Our interest is whether we can confidently think of an auditory cortical, somatosensory cortical, or visual cortical explanation for his "dissociated" naming problem—the difference between his responsive and visual confrontation naming.

For our ship builder, sounds, sights, and sensation enter the brain like parts for assembly, with near-normal responses to the spoken word. Listening seemed his relative strength, although other domains of his cortical function went either awry or, more likely, couldn't compensate when a task changed "mode"—e.g., the switch from responsive naming to visual confrontation naming.

*

Let me remind the reader where we ended chapter seven, after arrival at primary (core) auditory cortex. I'll cut and paste to help the memory: ". . . what seems perfectly unique in the primate and human brain is the exaggerated cortical territory between (beyond) so-called unimodal association areas—e.g., unimodal belt and parabelt connections lead afield from the core, and very far afield from the parabelt . . ." Here's a more comprehensive comment from researchers (Kaas et al., 1999b):

> Multimodal integration and cognitive influences on auditory percept formation are realized through connections of the parabelt with heteromodal and supramodal cortices.

To ask "what's in an anomia?" as opposed to "what's in a name?" is to entertain a Hughlings-Jacksonian idea inspired by a book on origins published in London in 1859: the (evolutionary) undevelopment of multimodality.

The Flechsigian tertiary field described by terms like "multimodal," "heteromodal," or "supramodal" cortex is where otherwise discrete sensory systems converge in a kind of interference pattern. (My dictionary says that an interference pattern happens when two or more amplitudes of coherent waves intersect.) We can only surmise that the intersection or interference of sensory-data streams happens somewhere (maybe many places) in the second of Wernicke's two large brain areas of functional significance–somewhere, that is, where the temporal, parietal, and occipital lobes "meet." As said earlier, exact localization is not our interest.

One wonders whether identifying solitary points of intersection would be suspect anyway.

10.

A Problem With Naming, Part II

I promised a second case. I return to my copy of Goodglass and Kaplan. To re-state what we've said: in general, a problem with responsive naming tends to be as severe as a problem in visual confrontation naming in aphasia, but with exceptions.

A 21 year-old male Vietnam veteran, an American, had been injured nine months before his presentation. A mortar shell fragment penetrated his brain. He had a right hemiparesis and a language problem. Regarding the latter, we have a snapshot, which I've edited (this is at six months after presentation, or 15 months after his injury; he somewhat improved over more than a year):

> Examiner: You were in the army?
> Patient: Special forces . . .
> Examiner: What did you do?
> Patient: Boom.
> Examiner: I don't understand.
> Patient: 'Splosions.

He scored in the 80th percentile in responsive naming (not bad) and just above the 40th percentile in visual confrontation naming (not good). To be more specific about the 80th-percentile score (unfortunately, we don't have the raw results), the veteran either responded haltingly to many questions or failed outright to answer two of these ten:

> What do we tell time with?
> What do you do with a razor?
> What do you do with soap?
> What do you with a pencil?
> What do we cut paper with?
> What color is grass?
> What do we light a cigarette with?
> How many things in a dozen?
> What color is coal?
> Where do you go to buy medicine?

Was his relative success due to brevity of acceptable answers? A word, just one, suffices in each case.

His writing was as sparse, like his monosyllabic "boom."

He could read, we're told. There's another portion of the Boston Diagnostic Aphasia Examination related specifically to reading aloud. In this subtest, the veteran scored in the 60th percentile–which means that he successfully articulated just two of ten sentences. I don't know which two he accomplished. Here are examples of somewhat complex statements to be vocalized:

> They heard him speak on the radio last night.

> The lawyer's closing argument convinced them.

Here are examples of simpler sentences:

You know how.

Limes are sour.

As said, we don't have raw results, so we don't know whether he succeeded with the terse or more complex items or whether he had problems with both. It's possible that the flow of longer sentences, their narrative quality, the past tense of the verbs, or some other idiosyncrasy made them easier to read for him. I can also see how "know how" could cause a reader to stumble into a paraph"r"asia such as "know ow" or "how now."

In the last chapter, we referred to multimodality involving the nonfrontal brain. What modes occupy the frontal and prefrontal brain?

*

Among discussions regarding what happens in naming and anomia, I find A.R. Luria compelling (Luria, 1972, also 1973 and 1980). He asks us to consider two surprisingly quirky questions that we might ask a patient or ourselves—these amount to a blend between a test of responsive naming and of reading. Example one:

When winter came, the streets were covered with _____.

Example two:

I went out to buy a _____.

What's the difference between the two, if any?

The answer to the first sentence completion task, to me, isn't obviously "snow." It could be "frost" or "ice" or (in the spirit of a writer like Tolstoy at wartime) "the life blood of Moscow." The second question more clearly introduces the problem of choice in *both* questions, since finding the right word is "indeterminate" (Luria's word) especially in the second instance. He explains further, "you simply need more information about the particular circumstances in order to select the right word from the storehouse of memory" (Luria, 1972). To me, word finding and naming always involves choice and always is indeterminate in some sense. What color is grass? Well, it depends. Brown is possible, based on experience in the lethal heat of summer.

We're in a position to appreciate a passage from Luria that I'll divide into three parts.

First part: *"It would be wrong to imagine that the naming of an object results from the simple manifestation of the established association between the image and the particular unique name"* (Luria, 1980). One has to agree. Luria refers to the kinds of elementary associations invoked in the ten questions of the responsive naming test. Naming isn't only a reflexive recall of cognitive connections. A person can perform rather well at such tasks without revealing the problem in an anomia. In severe aphasias, of course, even basic associations are lost—in which case, responsive and visual confrontation test results will correlate, and neither amounts to a good percentile score.

Second part; these sentences follow immediately after the one just quoted: *"As a rule, when we see an object (especially if we are not very familiar with it), not just a single name comes to mind, but a whole series of associations in which the particular object is enveloped. When we name an object we must select from these possible alternatives one association, inhibit all the rest . . .[.]"* Wait a minute.

"Inhibit"? It's easy enough to envision a multimodal area as a locale of assimilation, say, of primary sensory modalities which don't connect directly with each other in humans and primates—we basically characterized supra/hetero-modal processing as assimilation in the last chapter.

Then there's the word "enveloped." The associations in question aren't localizable to the dominant hemisphere. Recall that Wernicke believed memories to be everywhere in the brain—and who can dispute the possibility? But naming and dominant hemispheric function could be fundamentally related to each other because the envelopes (not their contents) develop there—at least when we attempt to use language for internal or externally directed purposes.

Third part: "*[. . . inhibit all the rest] . . . and thus, in fact, carry out an operation analogous to that taking place during differentiation.*" Differentiation in the context of Luria's discussion stands in counterpoint to generalization, the tendency for names to refer to some abstract or common property, as in the word "shoulder." It could be part of a human being, of a road, or a transitive act of getting through a crowd.

*

But, but, however, and yet: there's a problem, and I've partly created it. Recall the analogy of five people entering a building through separate doors, from chapter five.

I said that the five people never meet: crisp, red, fresh, sweet, firm. Yet somehow we construct the name or thought of an apple.

Do we now have to add an inhibition, a sixth sense that intones, "it's not a pear"?

Or, with respect to "mom," in addition to coo, brown eyes, flowery, milky, soft, do we now add a stark negation such as "precisely not someone else"?

Is *that* what frontal and prefrontal processing accomplishes? Do its "modes" include selection, inhibition, and even negation?

11.

Frontal Sparing?

Years ago, I reviewed a book by "neuroanthropologist" Terrence Deacon in which I learned about a syndrome first reported in New Zealand (Williams et al., 1961) and Germany (Beuren et al., 1962). Looking at my copy of Deacon now, I see that I double underlined a sentence about the syndrome on his page 269: "Both postmortem analysis and MRI analysis have revealed brains with a reduction of the entire posterior cerebral cortex, but a sparing of the cerebellum and frontal lobes, and perhaps even an exaggeration of cerebellar size" (Deacon, 1997). Back then, I had poked into the background literature, just a bit. The 1961 and 1962 papers talked about a combination of mental retardation and supravalvular aortic stenosis in children without much mention about their brains; we've learned since that those brains resemble isolated frontal lobe preparations, because much of the rest of the brain doesn't develop normally.

The 1962 paper by Beuren et al. described four children, ages 5½ to 10, three of whom had Wechsler IQ's in the 40's and 50's (normal being roughly 100). The authors wrote a lovely thing about their patients: "All have the same kind of friendly nature–they love everyone, are loved by everyone, and are very charming." A folded xerox of Beuren's paper is still in my copy of Deacon, between pages 268 and 269. Next to Beuren's name, I scrawled to myself, "Read more about this."

Williams syndrome, as it came to be known *sans* attribution to Beuren, is a homeobox genetic defect linked to chromosome seven. (For "homeobox" read: a sequence of genes having to do with embryologic development of the brain and other body parts.) Williams-Beuren brains exhibit relative preservation of anterior cortical volume, but *less* frontal volume when compared to a normal, age-matched controls; mesial temporal volume is also relatively preserved, with slightly *more* temporal volume compared to controls. The neocerebellum has a larger estimated surface area than controls (Bellugi et al., 2000).

To my eye, Deacon—I've now turned to his page 273—goes a bit crazy about the implications of the anatomy: "Williams syndrome provides a distorted mirror image of the genetic changes that must underlie the human symbolic bias. The underdevelopment of much of the brain but sparing of the frontal cortex and cerebellum . . . has given these two structures greater control over all cognitive processes. The effect is to exaggerate the bias to learn symbolic associations, even though the capacity to learn nonsymbolic associations is severely impaired."

Hold it.

Rewind.

*

We've said that primate and human brains differ from other animal brains because of certain exaggerated cortical territories, including multimodal cortex at the interface between occipital, temporal and parietal lobes posteriorly and, anteriorly, the prefrontal cortex rostral to the primary motor cortex. An anatomical difference, so Deacon's surmise goes, *must* be responsible for that which makes us human—i.e., symbolic more than non-symbolic (whatever that distinction supposedly means), linguistic as opposed to non-linguistic (ditto: whatever that difference is), proactive as opposed to reactive, charming as opposed to tedious, or what have you.

Says who?

Why *must* it be that relative sparing of prefrontal cortices equals, for example, an ability to symbolize or even to be charming? It's also plausible that the enlarged cerebellar hemispheres in Williams-Beuren syndrome could also be responsible for uniquely human traits. An argument why it *must* be so would enlist the same logic as Deacon's.

I ended the last chapter by asking, "Is *that* what frontal and prefrontal processing accomplishes?" A generous person might allow that I was partly right about the editing, selecting, inhibiting, even negating functions of prefrontal cortex. If I were encyclopedic, I'd add to the length of this book with scads of corroboration, starting probably with *de rigueur* talk about the case of Phineas Gage, whom I will not discuss. Instead, let's respond to a critic who asks, a tad belligerently, "at the end of the day, you don't know what the frontal lobes do, do you?" Candid answer: in fact, I don't presume to know, but I've got a trump card.

The nice thing about anatomy is that it's what it is. Anatomy doesn't change in the course of my lifetime or of the next generation's; we simply learn more about the anatomy that exists. In the next three chapters, I'm curious to discuss absolute basics of how the brain's lobes connect with each other, especially front to back. The essentials of my review date to Theodor Meynert of the Austro-Hungarian empire.

But, first, what is the exceedingly rare entity of Williams-Beuren syndrome . . . in more clinical detail than Deacon provides? In a report of semi-structured interviews with Williams-Beuren adolescents and adults, several responded to a stock question ("tell me about the favorite moment in your life") along these lines: "Being here [*at the semi-structured interview!*] is the best thing that ever happened to me." We read that "a strong drive toward social interaction makes up an important and distinctive part of the [Williams-Beuren] behavioral phenotype" (Jones et al., 2000).

Even in the context of overall mental retardation and developmental delay, there's something savant-like and enchanting about their conversational language, their fascination with the look of others as conversation happens, their buoyant affect, etc., all specifically in association with their frontally spared brains. Or perhaps in association with their spared mesial temporal lobes. Or perhaps with their large cerebellar hemispheres.

*

It's a bedside test that many clinicians use, especially in the evaluation of a dementia: "name all the animals you can think of in one minute." The number of animals named is the result of interest in the challenge (if you get to 15 different animals, you're more or less not Alzheimerian), but what's to be made of these responses from adolescents with Williams-Beuren syndrome (Bellugi et al, 2000)?

> . . . tiger, owl, sea lion, zebra, hippopotamus, turtle, lizard, reptile, frog, beaver, giraffe, chihuahua . . .

or:

> . . . ibex, whale, bull, yak, zebra, puppy, kitten, tiger, koala, dragon . . .

Early word and language acquisition is delayed in Williams-Beuren, but by school age—and especially after age 11—facility with words and a "proclivity" for low-frequency names emerges.

Despite adroitness with words, visuospatial praxis is problematic: a drawing of a house yields no sense of any building. Even in the verbal description of a spatial relationship (two 13 year-olds are shown an apple in a bowl), responses included "the bowl is in the apple" and "the apple is around the bowl." Yet, in the rather demanding Benton Face Recognition test, in which one is shown a "target" face and must select other face photos at different angles and under various lighting conditions to match the target, 16 subjects with Williams-Beuren syndrome (ages 8-22 years) performed nearly on par with normal controls, with a mean percent of correct face matches of roughly 93%. Then, there's the joy of simply listening to a 14-year old talking about herself; her IQ is 49: "You're looking at a professional book writer. My books will be filled with drama, action, and excitement. Everyone will want to read them. I'm going to write books, page after page, stack after stack." Delightful.

Back to a ponderous Deacon, now on his page 427: ". . . the hypersociality of Williams syndrome patients, and their intense monitoring and solicitation of others' responses in social interactions, may also be understood not just as a function of modified affect but as a shift in cognitive style, in which an exaggerated prefrontal bias may lead to an exaggerated reliance on symbolic prediction of others' behaviors." Human neocortex—by which I mean all cortex with the exception of archicortex (hippocampus) and paleocortex (primary olfactory cortex)—*and* connections of neocortex to diverse points constitute an estimated 80% of human brain volume (Shepherd, 1998). In medical school teaching today, though a change is almost certainly imminent, we don't address connectivity with sophistication. As a consequence, a throwback argument emerges like Deacon's, one that unavoidably raises the possibility of pseudo-localization: *what if* there's no discrete locale for symbolic capacity any more than there are clear demarcations for Broca's or Wernicke's areas?

Likewise, could disconnection theory as advocated by Wernicke's intellectual descendants mislead us into thinking that syndromes result from clipping this wire or those wires, as if the wires in question were readily localizable? In fairness, both the disconnection theorists and our neuroanthropologist would acknowledge that so-called human functions (e.g., Deacon's "symbolic bias") involve swaths of cortex in the front and back, and maybe subcortical structures as well–in other words, dispersed brain locales, not without their interesting connections between each other.

So, how to discuss connectivity in a teachable and meaningful way?

Is language and symbolic capacity frontal? Yes. *H. sapiens* and the 14-year-old professional book writer seem to be cases in point, like legal precedents that could admit further argument. Language and symbolic capacity are also parietal, temporal, occipital–perhaps limbic, thalamic, and hypothalamic (viz., subcortical), too.

How a brain coheres is the issue.

12.

Connectivity I: Hodology

The word may soon become obsolete; to be honest, it hasn't been commonly used anyway in my experience teaching neuroanatomy: "hodology" (from the Greek, *hodos*, a path, akin to the Latin *tractus*) may well yield to "connectome" or "connectomics." We'll learn, we hope, about relevant tractography by way of the human connectome project, which is ongoing as I write these sentences in 2018.

In the mean time, you can Google "hodology" to learn about hodographs in meteorology and mathematics or about "hodological space" in psychology, the latter championed by Kurt Levin (1890-1947), whose concept of social connectedness involved more than personal interactions at points in time, but rather invoked bounded networks of those whom we meet, perhaps casually if not randomly, in a long sequence of phases in life. Lewin, it's been said, was interested in "the push and pull of forces" in social contexts which he described by way of "Jordan curves" (Google that term, too, if you like) which he would draw anywhere, "on blackboards, scraps of paper, in the dust, or in the snow," which his students affectionately called "Lewin's eggs" or "Lewin's bathtubs" (Hunt, 2004). Connectivity as a bathtub: *that's* a concept that I'd love to see introduced into neuroanatomical teaching, but I won't live that long.

This chapter's aim is simple, so let me say what I intend in neuroanatomic-ese, a supremely parochial language, then I'll elaborate, and I'll be as brief as I can possibly be.

Autochthonous (local), short, or "U" association fibers–"association fiber" is Theodor Meynert's term–are intimately associated with long association fibers connecting, for example, frontal and occipital lobes– which is to say, the longitudinal extent of cortex. Long association fibers can be dissected and are well known to anatomists, but the blunt postmortem dissection that reveals them "strip[s] superficial layers of fibers to visualize deeper ones, destroying their anatomical relation" (ffytche and Catani, 2005).

*

If you understood the last paragraph, go ahead to the next chapter. If you didn't, let me explain myself.

*

If we were to describe the brain not by surface anatomy, not by lobes as viewed on the lateral or medial surfaces of an intact hemisphere, but rather from the inside out, how would the anatomy look? A thought experiment might enlist the following "virtual" dissection.

Imagine that you hold a gross specimen, an entire cerebral hemisphere, in your hand. As we do in lab, we scalpel cut at the level of the midbrain, so that the brainstem and cerebellum connected to it fall away. Then, let's (conceptually) remove diencephalon, specifically all four tiers that are neatly separated layers in a developing brain: *epithalamus*, *thalamus* (in embryology, the "dorsal thalamus"), *subthalamus* (including the rostral extent of the midbrain tegmentum; so, we remove basal grey matter like substantia nigra and all grey structures in its vicinity, including globus pallidus and others, as well as some white matter like the lenticular fasciculus ["H2"], ansa lenticularis, and thalamic fasciculus ["H1"]–the latter three tracts connect globus pallidus to thalamus), and all of *hypothalamus*.

If you insist that your interest is just neocortex, then you could also rid yourself of grey-matter structures of the corpus striatum (putamen and caudate), but you spare the internal capsule; you'd rid yourself, too, of all of the archicortical hippocampus and maybe even that nubbin in humans, the paleocortical olfactory cortex, and maybe amygdala as well. What's left is all neocortex.

Now we dissolve all neuronal cell bodies, just them (not their axons), then we look at the white matter that remains. An analogy that I have in mind–as a reminder, this is purely a virtual dissection–is to visualize the frame structure of, say, the Statue of Liberty by evaporating all that we externally see of it: the robe, the torch, the crown, the tablet of law held in the left arm, etc.

In a crude first-pass view, we'd reveal lengthwise beams spanning from front to back in the hemisphere.

From top to bottom in that hemisphere, beam-wise, we see: the *cingulum* (not the cingulate gyrus, because we dissolved its neurons), the *subcallosal bundle* (also known as the *superior occipitofrontal fasciculus*, which intersects the corpus callosum, which passes from side to side), the *superior longitudinal fasciculus*, and the *inferior occipitofrontal fasciculus* (which passes through the extreme capsule). For good measure, there's also an *inferior longitudinal fasciculus*, which passes from back not quite all the way forward–if cortex were present, we'd notice that it passes from occipital to temporal lobe, not to frontal lobe.

That amounts to six principle length-wise beams. The first three intersect, more or less orthogonally, to the fibers of the *corona radiata*.

Vertically, we notice three main struts: from front to back, the *orbitofrontal fasciculus*, the *uncinate fasciculus*, and the *vertical occipital fasciculus*.

From hemisphere across to the other hemisphere, the *corpus callosum* is thick and enormous. We bisected it, because we were interested just in one hemisphere.

*

There's a nomenclature issue that brings to mind the complaint raised against blunt dissection just a moment ago. The superior longitudinal fasciculus–which is very long, and curves inferiorly, heading towards the beam that we've identified as the inferior longitudinal fasciculus–goes by an alternate name. It's also called the *arcuate fasciculus*–"arcuate," we remind ourselves quickly, refers only to something that *bends*. The arcuate fasciculus doesn't "arch" between the putative areas of Wernicke and Broca. To say so is an oversimplification (Bernal and Ardila, 2009).

Then again, the six beams and three struts that we've identified are also simplifications that give rise to possible misconceptions of this type:

From front to back,

> *cingulum* "goes" from parolfactory area to entorhinal cortex
>
> *subcallosal bundle* (also known as the *superior occipitofrontal fasciculus*) "goes" from frontal to temporal and occipital lobes
>
> *superior longitudinal fasciculus* (also known as *arcuate fasciculus*) "goes" between Wernicke's and Broca's areas

> *inferior occipitofrontal fasciculus* (which intersects the extreme capsule) "passes" between frontal and occipital lobes
>
> *inferior longitudinal fasciculus* "passes" between occipital and temporal lobes

From top of bottom,

> *orbitofrontal fasciculus* "extends" between superior and inferior frontal lobe
>
> *uncinate fasciculus* "extends" between temporal to frontal lobes
>
> *vertical occipital fasciculus* "goes" between superior and inferior occipital lobe

The ironic quotation marks and even the blah verbs I use (go, pass, extend) are intentional: I'm tentative to teach hodology, because we just don't know enough yet about what the (often bidirectional) connections mean, never mind the little we know about shorter "U" fibers associated with each of these grossly dissectible paths. It's not that the above statements aren't anatomically correct—in fact, you can find them corroborated in standard textbooks going back decades. For me, however, there's a disconnection between a basic understanding of the brain's white-matter framework and any association with cortical function.

Going back to the frame-structure analogy, if you knew the interior struts and beams of the Statue of Liberty, you could visualize the green-hued statue itself as it stands in New York Harbor or, no less justifiably, you could also envision the Eiffel Tower in Paris, since the frameworks are similar and are both products of Gustave Eiffel's consistent imagination (Lidwell et al., 2010).

Put differently: in the absence of correlations—i.e., advanced hodology plus histological parcellations, plus topological reconstructions (since cortical folding is a challenge to understanding which parts of cortex activate either at rest or in a task—note that a good two-thirds of cortex lies within sulcal depths), plus clinical correlations, etc.—hodology feels like a curio of an academic past. I do think, however, that hodological basics reviewed in the last several pages call attention to the massive connectivity of frontal brain to all lobes—which is to say, to everywhere in the human brain.

But even Ernest Aubertin suspected as much when he applied a spatula to the exposed frontal brain of his patient on April 4, 1861.

13.

Connectivity II: Projection and Association

What follows isn't a quiz about the one projection-fiber pathway that medical students recall even if they've forgotten all other neuroanatomy. The corticospinal tract, I'll assume, is familiar enough. But I do have a question: what is it, anatomically? It "projects" (Meynert's term) from cortex, but its terminus is not cortical.

A projection fiber differs from an association fiber that arises from cortex in a hemisphere to arrive at other cortex in the same hemisphere; there are short and long association fibers, as we outlined in the last chapter. And there's another kind of association fiber that connects across the two hemispheres—if the connection happens between "like" cortical areas (e.g., ipsilateral frontal to contralateral frontal), one refers to a *homotopic* interhemispheric association fiber. Commissural fibers in the corpus callosum are interhemispheric and, as a rule of thumb, homotopic.

Alternatively, if the lobe of origin in one hemisphere differs from its lobar destination in the opposite hemisphere (e.g., contralateral parietal to ipsilateral frontal), one refers to a *heterotopic* interhemispheric association fiber. Though I use the singular "fiber," we're talking about tracts which either can be demonstrated in careful anatomical dissection or which are obvious, as in the case of corpus callosum or the anterior commissure.

Not all projection fibers arise from cortical sites. Let's describe the "last mile" (as telecommunication providers call the final connection to your house) from medial geniculate nucleus/body to primary auditory cortex, otherwise known as the koniocortical core in the transverse gyri of Heschl. Fibers project from medial geniculate nucleus; they course laterally; they encircle the lateral geniculate nucleus of the visual pathway, then, at the very low border of the putamen in the lentiform nucleus, they penetrate the descending fibers of the internal capsule and ascend due northward (superiorly) to temporal lobe. So, fibers originating from medial geniculate nucleus *project*. And cortex projects back: the final mile isn't a one-way connection, since parabelt connects reciprocally with thalamus–not only medial geniculate nucleus, but also medial pulvinar (Kaas et al., 1999b).

A different example: what about projections from prefrontal motor areas to subcortical sites in basal ganglionic connectivity? For a student interested in the basal ganglia, there's a mantra that one intones in sleep, that a frontal cortical area having to do with movement connects with a specific striatal locale, then to a pallidal one, thence to a thalamic one. The circuit closes with a projection from a thalamic nucleus related to movement back to the cortical site of origin–i.e., the place, even the neuron, at the start of the loop. What's the projection neuron in this scenario? There are two: from cortex to striatum and from thalamus to cortex. In effect, the above is an instance of a projection pathway serving basically the function of an association fiber from a cortical area/neuron back to itself.

*

One can teach neuroanatomy long enough, using antique tricks to get students to recall that or this, that one enters a rut. Consider how I've taught the connection(s) between cerebral cortex and cerebellar cortex—more specifically, left cortex and right cerebellum.

I have a slim, German textbook with good illustrations (Kahle, 1986) which I've consulted for years. Even knowing that some of its information is obsolete, I use it as a touchstone: areas of cortex (left frontal and left temporal) project via the left internal capsule towards ipsilateral, left cerebral peduncle, Kahle says—so I parrot Kahle.

The central third of that (left) peduncle or crus cerebri largely contains corticospinal fibers destined to form the left pyramid, but the medial third contains a frontopontine tract (so-called Arnold's bundle); the lateral third contains a temporopontine tract (so-called Türck's bundle). The bundles of Arnold (medial) and Türck (lateral) myelinate later in development than the corticospinal tract (Engelhardt, 2013). Frontopontine and temporopontine projections end at pontine nuclei ipsilaterally; frontopontine fibers terminate more rostrally than temporopontine fibers do.

After synapsing at pontine nuclei, essentially all fibers cross the brainstem's midline in the pons (*pons*, Latin for bridge, as in the word "pontiff," a bridge between god and man). Axons arising from pontine nuclear neurons comprise the large middle cerebellar peduncles on either side. Projections that have arisen originally from left cortex, via right middle cerebellar peduncle, terminate mainly in the right cerebellar hemisphere as mossy fibers, though some project bilaterally, also as mossy fibers, in the midregion of cerebellar vermis.

I've taught all the above—and left cortex does (roughly) connect to right cerebellar hemisphere as described. "That's how cortex talks to contralateral cerebellum," I glibly say. *Talks*? Isn't the verb too . . . colloquial? Moreover, do I miss the fundamental point? As a colleague of mine says, there's *cum laude* teaching, then there's a *summa* way. A person should choose how to perform.

*

Based on studies in the rhesus monkey (Schmahmann, 1996), much—probably not all—of left cortex maps onto left pontine nuclei (motor/premotor and dorsolateral prefrontal, parietal, and superior temporal cortices clearly do, according to multiple sources); there's "a mosaic" of left cortical terminations in the left pons. In cats, "distinct" projections from left auditory cortex end in left pons in this cerebrocerebellar pathway (Nieuwenhuys, 2008). Even some fibers of *the corticospinal tract* synapse at the pontine nuclei, and will descend no further caudally (Brodal, 1981). Corticospinal collaterals map onto pontine nuclei maintaining somatotopy.

In turn, efferent cerebello-cortical axons arising, for example, from the dentate nucleus project, via ventral and dorsomedial thalamic nuclei, back to what we've previously called multimodal cortical areas, including prefrontal cortex and intraparietal areas. In the last projection, which closes a cortico-*cerebellar*-cortical loop, aren't we describing a kind of association pathway linking cortical locales back to cortical locales, as we saw in the case of basal ganglia connectivity?

A lesson to consider, maybe a *summa* point, is as follows: you could discuss, as we have,

>... thalamus to cortex, or

>cortex to thalamus (it's a two-way "final mile"), or

>cortex and striatum, or

>cortex and pons, or

pons and cerebellum, or

cerebellum back to cortex, or

cortex and other cortex, or

a specific cortical locale and that very cortex itself . . .

and, all the while, projections seem more and more like associative pathways. There are many implications of the statement, not the least of which being a prediction that locales associated with each other will activate together *of course.*

In the sense I invoke, "association" isn't necessarily a wire or discrete fiber. I mean something more along the lines of: actions that cohere in time and in anatomical space.

14.

Connectivity III: An Old Paper

When you're wrestling with a subject not for the sake of an exam, but rather because you want to understand more about it (the subject, not the exam), there's a strategy that proves useful on occasion.

Don't assume that the latest issue of *Nature Neuroscience* or similar periodical will yield the insight you seek.

Be different, rear guard, even Luddite. Go as far back as you need to go; find a relevant and intelligent paper whose methods you actually understand and can articulate for yourself. Print it on paper, then weigh into it. Start to think or write, mainly for yourself.

Our problem is how to think about language as an activity of spatially discrete locales. We discuss connectivity, because neurons do connect for a fact, but it's a more and more intricate concept in the 21st century, as we'll discuss in our second-to-last chapter. To peek ahead, in what way is connectivity "a history of neuronal coactivation" (Gordon et al., 2016)? More later.

For now, what's "a connection," aside from a line between dots?

After we arrive at a primary sensory cortex (we've focused on the auditory pathway), what really happens . . . in what sequence . . . or: is there a sequence? Let's say that it won't suffice to answer, as we've heard before, that *primary projection areas now send their connections primarily to the immediately adjacent association cortex (parakoniocortex).*

*

A paper that I appreciate, because its method is straightforward and its writing elegant, dates to 1970 (Jones and Powell, 1970). The authors studied rhesus monkeys. They dissected tiny areas of pia mater off the cortical surface, causing avascular necrosis of the grey matter beneath; there was rather little damage to white matter beneath the grey matter. After 7-14 days, they fixed the brains, sectioned them into 25-micron-thick slices, then stained those using established techniques (e.g., Nauta staining). They were interested to learn the distribution of axonal degeneration in a hemisphere after lesions of specific cortical locales in that hemisphere. One could call the methodology quaint, but that's why I've chosen the paper.

Slight problem: the primary auditory cortical surface hides deep in the lateral (Sylvian) fissure in rhesus monkeys as in humans, so the authors couldn't be sure that they wouldn't damage parietal cortex superiorly or the superior temporal gyrus inferiorly in their attempt to lesion. They probably did inflict damage in what we'd identify today as belt or parabelt. Their honesty speaks to how fastidiously they wanted to isolate only primary sensory areas. Primary somatosensory cortex and primary visual cortex were easier targets.

Despite the inaccessibility of Heschl's gyri, a consistent pattern emerged for auditory, somatosensory, and visual projections due to allegedly primary cortical lesions: "each primary area projects to an local area in the same lobe *and* to a portion of premotor cortex in the frontal lobe." Then they followed the paths laid down before them, where degenerated axons appeared after their microsurgeries. If a first, discrete lesion close to primary auditory cortex resulted in white-matter degeneration underlying a larger superior temporal area, then they lesioned the larger superior temporal area. The first lesion resulted, as we just read, in premotor axonal degeneration in specific *frontal* areas; the (second) larger superior temporal lesion also resulted in prefrontal axonal degeneration in different, more widespread frontal areas, specifically orbitofrontal cortex, frontal operculum, and frontal pole (Brodmann's areas 8, 9, 10, and 12).

Likewise, a lesion of primary somatosensory cortex resulted in axonal degeneration in Brodmann's area 5, posterior to (and abutting) primary sensory cortex, but also in the area of primary motor cortex. Then a lesion in area 5 resulted in degeneration in nearby area 7 in the inferior parietal lobule, but also area 6, which is the supplementary motor cortex anterior to primary motor cortex. Note that areas 5-7 are not at all contiguous: 5 and 7 are parietal; 6 is rostral and frontal.

If it seems that sensory projections might converge in prefrontal lobe exclusively, think again. Somatosensory, visual, and auditory convergence also happens in the area of the superior temporal sulcus (Brodmann's area 22, with extension posteriorly and superiorly to areas 39 and 40, in area of the inferior parietal lobule). The superior temporal sulcus separates superior temporal gyrus from middle temporal gyrus; it's the first sulcus inferior to the Sylvian fissure in temporal lobe.

There's more to the paper as we'll see, but what the authors termed "double projection" from a primary sensory area both to immediate-neighborhood cortex *and* to frontal lobe–to frontal and temporal lobes in the case of their study of primary auditory cortex–makes one rethink stepwise processing. The authors seem to follow a single trail, at first. In their somatosensory study, they lesioned primary sensory cortex, then adjacent area 5, but the trail had already scattered to rostral points (to primary motor cortex). They also lesioned primary motor cortex to find axonal changes under the frontal eye field and both primary and secondary sensory cortices–in other words, a good chunk of both frontal and parietal cortices. Their trail was dictated by where axons degenerated after lesions, but what if spatially separate brain areas could be observed to relate to each other, "cohere," or even coactivate based on other ways of looking at brains (see chapter 15)?

*

The authors were fundamentally curious to know in what ways sensory pathways converge. They concluded: "The most obvious regions of convergence are in the depths of the superior temporal sulcus (probably the homologue of areas 39 and 40 in man), at the frontal pole, and in orbito-frontal cortex of the frontal operculum."

What about olfaction? I'll paraphrase the authors to highlight how clever, even devious, their answer is: why not follow the auditory pathway (or visual or somatosensory ones)? Anyone can trace the olfactory pathway[1]; the authors back their way into that anatomy.

Recall the problem described in chapter five. How to bind CRISP, RED, FRESH, SWEET, FIRM? We can start with CRISP.

A discrete lesion close to primary auditory cortex resulted in degeneration underlying a larger superior temporal area, so the authors lesioned the larger superior temporal area. That led to axonal degeneration at the frontal pole, so they lesioned the frontal pole to find degeneration at the rostral cingulate gyrus, among other places. As auditory, visual, and somatosensory pathways begin to converge,

---

[1] In neuroanatomy lab, we follow a pathway from olfactory bulb and tract to a bifurcation of that tract at basal forebrain; the lateral olfactory stria enters pyriform cortex (it's small in humans as compared to other animals), periamygdaloid cortex, and parahippocampal gyrus–all of which are paralimbic.

connections ramify across cortex . . . eventually towards paralimbic and limbic locales (e.g., rostral cingulate, as we just said).

The cingulate gyrus, we recall, is also paralimbic, a different point of entry into limbic lobe.

The authors cite a transition zone, a simian homolog to area 35 in humans, "part of which adjoins the pyriform cortex and receives fibers from the olfactory pathway," the paralimic rest of which receives connections from auditory, visual, and somatosensory systems. The regions of convergence the authors identified (areas 39 and 40 in parietal lobe, at the superior extent of superior temporal gyrus; the frontal pole; orbitofrontal cortex at the frontal operculum) also project to limbic cortex, thence to hippocampus.

In other words, they account for FRESH smell in concert with CRISP, RED, and FIRM. Maybe they get partial credit for SWEET taste as well, since smell and taste occupy much the same sensory space.

*

Fine, there's a lot to be learned by tracing Meynert's association fibers hither and yon. What about language?

By the way, isn't it curious that the areas of sensory convergence are roughly Broca's and Wernicke's areas (if we think about the dominant hemisphere)?

15.

A Note on Dominance

This monograph is the second in a series of short publications whose goal is to address a certain kind of question that students ask from time to time. There are factual queries in abundance that textbooks answer, then someone wonders out loud, for example, "why do tracts cross the axial midline in neuroanatomy?" If the immediate answer is "because they do," then perhaps (such is my premise) there's something to ponder in a non-textbook format. The preceding chapters don't address "why is the left brain dominant for language in most people?" One wonders whether a different installment, yet another book, is necessary to frame a response, but a couple of pages will suffice today.

*

"Dominance" is a problematic word (if there's dominance, is there submission?), because one actually refers to lateralization of a function. But "lateralization" isn't perfect either, because there are ways in which asymmetry dominates in life. I write (as opposed to type), draw, shave, hammer, brush my teeth, throw etc. with my right hand; my parents and their parents were all righties; I kick with my right foot far better than with my left; if I position my right thumb over a distant object with both eyes open, then close my right eye, my thumb is very much off the distant target—not so if I close my left eye (I'm right-eye dominant). Right handedness and left hemispheric lateralization for language go together for the vast majority of both right-and left-handed persons. At a patient's bedside, if I see a right hemiparesis, I'm eager to examine a language problem; if I see a left hemiparesis, I'm very interested to learn if there's a syndrome of neglect.

(Lateralization of neural function isn't unique to humans. I read that there's left-hemispheric dominance in frogs, songbirds, and mice when they vocalize, and that roughly two-thirds of chimpanzees throw right handed [Corballis, 2003 and 2014]. I read with greater curiosity that in the zebrafish pineal complex or epithalamus there's a genetically determined neuronal asymmetry resulting in an asymmetrically large left habenular nucleus; inactivation of the left habenula causes zebrafish to freeze, not turn away, in response to threat [Concha et al, 2012].)

We shouldn't forget that even if a function lateralizes, there are still homotopic associative connections between the hemispheres via transcallosal fibers between hemispheres. In fact, there are academics who *explain* hemispacial neglect in relation to connections between homologous cortex. Right hemisphere (posterior parietal lobe) directs attention to both hemispaces, whereas left hemisphere (posterior parietal lobe) directs only to right hemispace. Right hemisphere compensates in the case of a left hemisphere lesion in terms of attention to right hemispace.

Right hemisphere lesions result in neglect of left hemispace, because the left hemisphere drives attention only to right hemispace. Here's a theory that's been advanced, with some data to support it: by way of transcallosal fibers, right hemisphere inhibits its homologous area in left hemisphere to a greater degree than left inhibiting right, so asymmetry in function results, with right hemisphere dominant for spatial awareness (Koch et al., 2011).

Is there an analogous argument in the verbal or linguistic domain? Left hemisphere (frontoparietal) drives language production and inhibits its homologous area(s) in right hemisphere to a greater degree than right inhibiting left, so asymmetry in function results, with left hemisphere dominant for language?

*

Or not.

As psychologist Martha Farah has written with delicious acidity in a different context, maybe "the ratio of critical data to hypotheses is probably too low to expect any immediate resolution . . . " (Farah, 1990).

*

But there's no stopping the hypothesizing academic. Consider a last morsel (Corballis, 2003):

> I argue that language evolved from manual gestures, gradually incorporating vocal elements. The transition may be traced through changes in the function of Broca's area. Its homologue in monkeys has nothing to do with vocal control, but contains the so-called "mirror neurons," the code for both the production of manual reaching movements and the perception of the same movements performed by others. This system is bilateral in monkeys, but predominantly left-hemispheric in humans, and in humans is involved with vocalization as well as manual actions.

The ten-page paper from which I quote is followed by 50 or so pages of "open peer commentary," not all of which is flattering, as one might imagine. My favorite title in the bunch of critical aftermath is: "A shrug is not a sentence."

It's true. You can't hear a shrug.

16.

Metaconnectivity

Our big story nears its end.

The little story of this chapter begins with an homage.

There are people I've met who can flat-out *teach*: they take a very complicated subject, and, within the first few sentences of what they write or, more often, when they speak, it's as if every fetter of difficulty falls away, and what's left standing is like a sculpture that's geometric in clarity and simplicity, but the shape engages the eye and mind completely. A number of these great teachers, unfortunately, have either retired and vanished or have died. Some still linger, though they're not always noticed. The point is: there aren't many of them. Rare birds and hens' teeth have been encountered more frequently. I invoke the spirit of that elite now, because we enter a subject that has always seemed to me more turgid than lucid.

*

This chapter about current-day functional MRI (fMRI) has seen several drafts on my computer, all of them deleted. In the worst one, I talked about terms bandied about today, such as a dorsal-attention, default, and frontoparietal networks, only to realize that subdivisions of these and others going by different names give a sense of a shifting map or one still in the making.

In a slightly better but still lousy draft, I talked about a rumor that Korbinian Brodmann's famous cytoarchitectural subdivisions, which we mentioned in chapter four, were based on just one human brain (Brodmann, 2006). It's probably true, as Margulies has observed (2017), that knowledge of human neuroanatomy in the 20th century has been based on extensive study of just a few brains. I compared the Brodmann rumor to the true story of a certain Russell A. Poldrack, who endured no less than 84 MRI sessions (during 33 of them, he reportedly "relaxed" with his eyes closed), to determine subject-specific, resting-state-functional-connectivity (RSFC) parcellations (Laumann et al., 2015). FYI: individual and group-based parcellations differ.

In a third try, I found myself talking about the biophysics of blood-oxygen-level-dependent (BOLD) signal fluctuations. Recall my story from chapter eight, about not speaking outside my ken. I won't.

All three drafts are gone; the single virtue of telling a story about them is: we now have two basic concepts in front of us, BOLD signal fluctuation and RSFC parcellation. The acronyms are less important, frankly, than the words "fluctuation" and "parcellation"–i.e., on the one hand, physiological variation in time as the brain does whatever it does; and, on the other, discrete units of neocortical space that have to do with each other somehow (perhaps mathematically), whether or not there are point-to-point axons known to connect them.

BOLD signal (Ogawa et al., 1990; Raichle and Mintun, 2006; Fox and Raichle, 2007) is a phenomenon whose nuances any non-physicist can appreciate. In a strong magnetic field, deoxygenated hemoglobin has a paramagnetic effect, but oxygenated hemoglobin doesn't. If neurons fire, they require oxygen and glucose. Localized blood flow and glucose consumption increase to a greater degree than oxygen consumed. Deoxygenated hemoglobin disrupts local MRI signal; that signal should *decrease* in an area of increased neuronal activity, but blood flow increases disproportionately, as does BOLD signal.

Three very elementary things fascinate me: 1. As one would expect, BOLD signal fluctuates in localities of brain (or in the brain as a whole); 2. You can quantify the fluctuation; and 3. BOLD signal fluctuation is analogous to noise, but not any noise (e.g., not white noise). There are websites that provide sound bites of different "colors" of noise. BOLD signal fluctuation has been characterized as "flicker" or "pink," and if the recordings I consulted are accurate, there's a subtle, audible difference between whiteness and flicker/pinkness. The latter noise is observed in a variety of complex, dynamic systems (Gilden et al., 1995).

With the above background alone, let's consider how BOLD signal and RSFC are used by researchers trying to describe a plain sense of mental life.

*

Here's a slightly edited paragraph that merits thought:

RSFC [resting state functional connectivity] relies on the observation that, in the absence of any task, spatially distant regions of cortex exhibit highly correlated patterns of blood oxygenation level-dependent (BOLD) activity . . . While the precise significance of RSFC is uncertain, accumulating evidence suggests that regions exhibiting RSFC correlations are also functionally coactive during tasks. In this view, these correlations observed during the resting state at least partly reflect the statistical history of regional coactivation (Gordon et al., 2016).

Note the following phrases as they relate to each other, from the beginning of the paragraph:

RSFC . . . in the absence of any task

spatially distant regions of cortex . . . highly correlated patterns of BOLD activity

In the assiduous fMRI study of just one brain, I'm not sure what Russell A. Poldrack thought about, recalled, imagined, or how his mood differed during his many sessions. But let's agree that there was no task he had to perform, aside perhaps from not falling asleep—or maybe he dozed from time to time. Why should there be RSFC, in which discrete cortical areas look alike in terms of BOLD activity (there were 616 parcels in total)?

What's a parcel, anyway?

A parcel is a bounded area in two dimensions. A boundary separates a cortical area that has the same pink/flicker noise value as some other grey matter region, all measurements having been made in the resting state (Cohen et al., 2008). Anywhere within a parcel, there should be homogeneous noise. (By the way, the story of 2D cortical maps is itself a fascinating saga; some didn't believe in their utility at first [Van Essen and Maunsell, 1980].)

So far, a take-home is that parcels defined by their respective noise profiles correlate across a brain at rest.[2]

---

[2] "Noise profile" is my coinage, used for simplicity. The technical term is $1/f$ noise, a temporal fluctuation that has a power density inversely proportional to the frequency—that is, power $\sim 1/f$ (Gilden et al., 1995).

Next, think about how these phrases relate to each other, from the end of the paragraph:

> regions exhibiting RSFC correlations . . . functionally coactive during tasks

> the resting state . . . the statistical history of regional coactivation

Russell A. Poldrack didn't spend all 84 sessions relaxing. In 51 sessions, he was put to work doing a variety of tests (some as simple as "open your eyes," "close your eyes"), all of them dutifully listed in a supplement to Laumann et al., 2015.

Anatomically separate areas of brain correlate both in a task and at rest so as to suggest their prior coactivation. Prior coactivation could predict what happens in the future, too. The resting state itself reflects "some combination of direct and indirect structural connectivity" (Gordon et al., 2016).

*

Does it occur to you that we have some redefinitions to consider? A parietal function isn't necessarily parietal; neither is a frontal one unequivocally frontal. And doesn't the phrase "some combination [of connectivities]" need more substance to it? Enter a paper that, when I read it, left me in no small state of wonderment (Goldman-Rakic and Schwartz, 1982).

Its methodology couldn't be simpler. Macaque monkeys were studied. Two different anterograde tracers were injected into two places, one left frontal and the other right parietal–both areas in the macaque are known to project to right prefrontal cortex (the left frontal projection crosses the midline via the corpus callosum). Just to be clear, the injections were: anterograde tracer A into left frontal lobe (Brodmann's area 9) and anterograde tracer B into right parietal lobe (Brodmann's area 7). Two days later, the monkeys were sacrificed; right prefrontal cortex was sectioned into 50-micron-thick coronal slices. Since the two tracers required different techniques to visualize terminal labeling, alternate coronal slices were processed separately, then camera lucida drawings of the slices were superimposed on each other, using local blood vessels as fiducial marks to get the images in register. The authors wanted to know the arrangement of the different terminal projections. They weren't sure that there would be any discernable order.

"Our major finding," they wrote,

> . . . is that callosal and associational axons ["associational" is Meynert's term, used here with reference to the terminal projections from ipsilateral parietal lobe] generally occupied mutually exclusive columnar territories, and, indeed, in areas of close convergence, columns of callosal axons alternated in short but regular sequences with those of associational input . . . Furthermore, reconstructions from serial sections . . . suggest that each fiber system is represented across the prefrontal cortex as a map of irregular stripes (Goldman-Rakic and Schwartz, 1982).

The widths of the stripes (or columns) varied, ~300 to 750 microns. But the stripes—the authors didn't fail to notice a similarity between their stripes and ocular dominance columns in visual neuroscience—traversed all six neocortical layers.

Sometimes, the stripes overlapped somewhat or even completely: "Thus, segregation of callosal and associational inputs in a rule that can be broken." Sometimes, there were unlabeled gaps between labeled stripes.

*

Here's a demonstration of what they found. "1" refers to a terminal field of tracer A; "2" refers to a terminal field of tracer B. There are six lines, representing six layers of prefrontal neocortex. But it should be added that overlaps ("1212") were occasionally more pronounced in specific layers–e.g., more overlap in layer VI as opposed to layer I. Also, "stripes" could appear more like triangles. In this schematic, I'll assume no difference in overlap between cortical layers, and the stripes are columnar:

```
11111222221212222222111    111122221111122221212111111122222211    11112222
11111222221212222222111    111122221111122221212111111122222211    11112222
11111222221212222222111    111122221111122221212111111122222211    11112222
11111222221212222222111    111122221111122221212111111122222211    11112222
11111222221212222222111    111122221111122221212111111122222211    11112222
11111222221212222222111    111122221111122221212111111122222211    11112222
```

In prefrontal cortex, there's representation of other brain areas in the same hemisphere and from the contralateral hemisphere. Gaps could represent projections from other territories not interrogated by the two anterograde tracers used in the experiment. In chapter 14, we looked at one experiment that begged a question about coherence of spatially discrete cortical areas. In the 1's and 2's above, we're schematizing coherence, which is akin to the types of correlations observed in RSFC study. We've concentrated on R.A. Poldrack in a condition of rest, but there's other study of individuals that reveals connectivity quite unique to persons (why would we expect otherwise?) and personal parcellations that blur in group-averaged data (Braga and Buckner, 2017).

We said that "fluctuation" and "parcellation" are the important words. So:

A stunning question comes to mind (Goldman-Rakic and Schwartz hint at it): who's to say that the above, highly schematic, columnar anatomy and, moreover, patterns of BOLD activity observed more than 35 years after the anterograde tracer study . . . to repeat, who's to say that all the above remains static or fixed over time . . . especially in a person's brain that, say, learns a language?

In metaconnectivity, wouldn't we expect something beyond static anatomy?

17.

Historical and Contemporary Conclusion

A Greek and Latin scholar wonders about how the epics of the ancient poet Homer, memorized by reciters contemporary to Homer and delivered in verbal performances to transmit knowledge to rapt audiences in that era, could be memorized in the first place:

> Why does *epic* oral storage of cultural information have to take narrative form? . . .
>
> The pleasures of rhythm are motor responses, they accompany actual motions of the body and mouth. This means that the process of recitation and of remembrance is itself a performance, a doing, a series of rhythmically co-ordinated actions. . . . [T]he preferred form of statement for memorisation will be one which describes "action." But acts can be performed only by "actors"; that is, by living agents who are "doing things." This can only mean that the preferred format for verbal storage in an oral culture will be the narrative of persons in action . . . (Havelock, 1982).

If we think of language as a skill learned *by doing*, then, thinking neurologically, we become curious about a relationship between, for example, motor cortex/cortices and memory . . . between doing and observing . . . between coordinated action and language itself. We mentioned in chapter 15 that action and language are hardly independent of each other, and treatises exist on the subject (e.g., Dehaene, 2009, reviewed in Miyawaki, 2010).

Language as a sensorimotor phenomenon is no revelation: we've always known it to be so. But the anatomic underpinnings of acts that are altogether sensory, motor, mnemonic, emotional, cultural, etc. are the stuff of many books written and still to be written.

I wonder, in retrospect, whether the title of this monograph is wrong somehow: "the 'frontal' brain and language" introduces a bias that maybe only the front matters. Nothing could be further from the truth, of course.

In self defense, I had history to tell that started, literally, in the frontal brain. It's quite a story, and I'll stick with it.

References

Books:

Aminoff, Michael J. *Brown-Séquard. A Visionary of Science*. New York: Raven Press, 1993.

Brodmann, Korbinian. *Brodmann's Localisation in the Cerebral Cortex*. [trans. Garey, LJ] New York: Springer, 2006.

Carpenter, Malcolm B. and Sutin, Jerome. *Human Neuroanatomy*. [8th ed.] Baltimore and London: Williams and Wilkins, 1983.

Deacon, Terrence W. *The Symbolic Species. The Co-evolution of Language and the Brain*. New York and London: W.W. Norton, 1997.

Dehaene, Stanislas. *Reading in the Brain. The Science and Evolution of a Human Invention*. New York: Viking, 2009.

Eggert, Gertrude H. *Wernicke's Works on Aphasia: A Sourcebook and Review*. The Hague: Mouton, 1977.

Farah, Martha J. *Visual Agnosia. Disorders of Object Recognition and What They Tell Us about Normal Vision*. Cambridge and London: MIT Press, 1990.

Finger, Stanley. *Origins of Neuroscience. A History of Explorations into Brain Function*. Oxford and New York: Oxford, 1994.

Finger, Stanley. *Minds Behind the Brain: A History of the Pioneers and their Discoveries*. New York: Oxford, 2000.

Goodglass, Harold and Kaplan, Edith. *The Assessment of Aphasia and Related Disorders.* [2nd ed.] Philadelphia: Lea and Febiger, 1983.

Havelock, Eric A. *The Literate Revolution in Greece and Its Cultural Consequences.* Princeton: Princeton University Press, 1982.

Hunt, Morton. *The Story of Psychology.* New York: Anchor, 1994.

Kahle, Werner. *Nervous System and Sensory Organs.* [3rd revised edition, trans. H.L. and A.D. Dayan, Volume 3 of Kahle W., Leonhardt H, Platzer W. *Color Atlas and Textbook of Human Anatomy*] Stuttgart and New York: Georg Thieme, 1986.

Lidwell, William, Holden Kritina, and Butler, Jill. *Universal Principles of Design.* Beverly, MA: Rockport, 2010. (See chapter entitled "Structural Forms.")

Locke, Simeon. *Mind. An Emergent Property.* Bloomington: Xlibris, 2014.

Luria, A.R. *Human Brain and Psychological Processes.* [trans. Haigh, B.] New York and London: Harper and Row, 1966.

Luria, A.R. *The Man with a Shattered World. The History of a Brain Wound.* [trans. Solotaroff, L.] Cambridge: Harvard University Press, 1972.

Luria, A.R. *The Working Brain. An Introduction of Neuropsychology.* [trans. Haigh, B.] New York: Basic Books, 1973.

Luria, Aleksandr Romanovich. *Higher Cortical Functions in Man.* [2nd ed., trans. Haigh, B.] New York: Basic Books, 1980.

McHenry, Lawrence C., Jr. *Garrison's History of Neurology.* Springfield: Charles C. Thomas, 1969.

Mesulam M.-Marsel. *Principles of Behavioral and Cognitive Neurology.* [2nd ed.] Oxford and New York: Oxford, 2000.

Nolte, John. *The Human Brain. An Introduction to Its Functional Anatomy.* [4th ed.] St. Louis: Mosby, 1999.

Shepherd, Gordon M [ed.] *The Synaptic Organization of the Brain.* [4th ed.] New York and Oxford: Oxford University Press, 1998. (See chapter 12, "Neocortex" by Douglas and Martin.)

*

Articles:

Anonymous. The University of Vienna, *British Medical Journal* 1874;2(713):282-283.

Anonymous. An introduction to the life and work of John Hughlings Jackson. *Medical History Supplement* 2007; (26): 3–34.

Bellugi U, Lichtenberger L, Jones W, Lai Z, St. George M. The neurocognitive profile of Williams syndrome: a complex pattern of strengths and weaknesses. *Journal of Cognitive Neuroscience* 2000;12 supplement 1:7-29.

Berker EA, Berker AT, Smith A. Translation of Broca's 1865 report: localization of speech in the third left frontal convolution. *Archives of Neurology* 1986;43:1065-1072.

Bernal B, Ardila A. The role of the arcuate fasciculus in conduction aphasia. *Brain* 2009;132:2309-2316.

Beuren AJ, Apitz J, Harmjanz D. Supravalvular aortic stenosis in association with mental retardation and a certain facial appearance. *Circulation* 1962;26:1235-1240.

Braga RM, Buckner RL. Parallel interdigitated distributed networks within the individual estimated by intrinsic functional connectivity. *Neuron* 2017;95:457-471.

Broca P. Perte de la parole, ramollisement chronique et destruction partielle du lobe antérieur gauche du cerveau [Loss of speech, chronic softening and partial destruction of the left anterior lobe of the brain]. *Bulletins de la Société d'Anthropologie* 1861a;2:235-238, available in translation in Wilkins, Robert H (ed.). *Neurosurgical Classics*. American Association of Neurological Surgeons, 1992, pp. 63-64.

Broca P. Remarks on the seat of the faculty of articulated language, following an observation of aphemia (loss of speech). *Bulletin de la Société Anatomique* 1861b;6:330-357, in translation by Christopher D. Green at http://psychclassics.yorku.ca/Broca/aphemie-e.htm.

Catani M, ffytche DH. The rises and falls of disconnection syndromes. *Brain* 2005;128:2224-2239.

Catani M, Mesulam M. The arcuate fasciculus and the disconnection theme in language and aphasia: history and current state. *Cortex* 2008;44:953-961.

Cohen AL, Fair DA, Dosenbach NUF, Miezin FM, Dierker D, Van Essen DC, Schlaggar BL. Defining functional areas in individual human brains using resting functional connectivity MRI. *NeuroImage* 2008;41:45-57.

Concha ML, Bianco IH, Wilson SW. Encoding asymmetry within neural circuits. *Nature Reviews Neuroscience* 2012;13:832-843.

Corballis MC. From mouth to hand: gesture, speech, and the evolution of right-handedness. *Behavioral and Brain Sciences* 2003;26:199-260. (I also quote from Carstairs-McCarthy A. A shrug is not a sentence—which can be found on p. 215 in this citation.)

Corballis MC. Left brain, right brain: facts and fantasies. *PLoS Biology* 12(1): e1001767. doi:10.1371/journal.pbio.1001767.

Dehaene S, Cohen L, Sigman M, Vinckier F. The neural code for written words: a proposal. *Trends in Cognitive Sciences* 2005;9:335-341.

Dronkers NF, Plaisant O, Iba-Zizen MT, Cabanis EA. Paul Broca's historic cases: high resolution MR imaging of the brains of Leborgne and Lelong. *Brain* 2007;130: 1432-1441.

Engelhardt E. Cerebrocerebellar system and Türck's bundle. *Journal of the History of the Neurosciences* 2013;22:353-365.

ffytche DH, Catani M. Beyond localization: from hodology to function. *Philosophical Transactions of the Royal Society* 2005;360:767-779.

Flechsig P. Developmental (myelogenetic) localisation of the cerebral cortex in the human subject. *Lancet* 1901;158 (issue 4077):1027-1029.

Fox MD, Raichle ME. Spontaneous fluctuations in brain activity observed with functional magnetic resonance imaging. *Nature Reviews Neuroscience* 2007;8:700-711.

Geschwind N. "The work and influence of Wernicke." In: *Boston Studies in the Philosophy of Science* (vol. IV), eds. Cohen, Robert S. and Wartofsky, Marx W. Dordrecht: D. Reidel Publishing, 1969, pp. 1-33.

Geschwind N. "Disconnection syndromes in animals and man." In: *Selected Papers on Language and the Brain: Boston Studies in the Philosophy of Science* (vol. XVI), eds. Cohen, Robert S. and Wartofsky, Marx W. Dordrecht and Boston: D. Reidel Publishing, 1974, pp. 106-231.

Gilden DL, Thornton T, Mallon MW. $1/f$ noise in human cognition. *Science* 1995;267:1837-1839.

Goldman-Rakic PS, Schwartz ML. Interdigitation of contralateral and ipsilateral columnar projections to frontal association cortex in primates. *Science* 1982;216:755-757.

Gordon EM, Laumann TO, Adeyemo B, Huckins JF, Kelley WM, Petersen SE. Generation and evaluation of a cortical area parcellation from resting-state correlations. *Cerebral Cortex* 2016;26:288-303.

Greenblatt SH. The major influences on the early life and work of John Hughlings Jackson. *Bulletin of the History of Medicine* 1965;39:346-376.

Harris LJ. Early theory and research on hemispheric specialization. *Schizophrenia Bulletin*; 1999;25:11-39.

Haymaker W, "Paul Emil Flechsig." In: Haymaker W and Baer, Karl A, eds. *Founders of Neurology: One Hundred and Thirty-Three Biographical Sketches*, pp. 31-35.

Hickock G, Houde J, Rong F. Sensorimotor integration in speech processing: computational basis and neural organization. *Neuron* 2011;69:407-422.

Imaizumi K, Lee CC. Frequency transformation in the auditory lemniscal thalamocortical system. *Frontiers in Neural Circuits* 2014 (July);8:doi: 10.3389/fncir.2014.00075.

Jackson JH. On a case of loss of power of expression: inability to talk, to write, and to read correctly after convulsive attacks. *British Medical Journal* 1866;2 (Nos. 291 and 299):92-94 and 326-330.

Jackson JH. The Croonian lectures on evolution and dissolution of the nervous system. *British Medical Journal* 1884;1(No. 1213):591-593.

Jones W, Bellugi U, Lai Z, Chiles M, Reilly J, Lincoln A, Adolphs R. Hypersociability in Williams syndrome. *Journal of Cognitive Neuroscience* 2000;12 supplement 1:30-46.

Kaas JH, Hackett TA. (1999a) 'What' and 'where' processing in auditory cortex. *Nature Neuroscience* 1999;2:1045-1047.

Kaas JH, Hackett TA, Tramo MJ. (1999b) Auditory processing in primate cerebral cortex. *Current Opinion in Neurobiology* 1999;9:164-170.

Koch G, Cercignani M, Bonnì S, Giacobbe V, Bucchi G, Versace V, Caltagirone C, Bozzali M. Asymmetry of parietal interhemispheric connections in humans. *Journal of Neuroscience* 2011;31:8967-8975.

Laumann TO, Gordon EM, Adeyemo B, Snyder AZ, Joo SJ, Chen MY, Gilmore AW, McDermott KB, Nelson SM, Dosenbach NUF, Schlaggar BL, Mumford JA, Poldrack RA, Petersen SE. Functional system and areal organization of a highly sampled individual human brain. *Neuron* 2015;87:657-670.

Margulies DS. Unraveling the complex tapestry of association networks. *Neuron* 2017;95:239-241.

Mathews PJ, Obler LK, Albert ML. Wernicke and Alzheimer on the language disturbances of dementia and aphasia. *Brain and Language* 1994;46:439-463.

Miyawaki E. C:\Evolve: [Review of Deacon T., *The Symbolic Species: The Co-Evolution of Language and the Brain* and Pinker S., *How the Mind Works*]. *The Yale Review* 1998;86(4):128-139.

Miyawaki E. By the Book. [Review of Dehaene S. *Reading in the Brain: The Science and Evolution of a Human Invention*]. *The Yale Review* 2010;98(4):140-153.

Ogawa S, Lee TM, Kay AR, Tank DW. Brain magnetic resonance imaging with contrast dependent on blood oxygenation. *Proceedings of the National Academy of Sciences* (United States) 1990;87:9868-9872.

Olry R, Haines DE. NEUROwords. Korbinian Brodmann: the Victor Hugo of cytoarchitectonic brain maps. *Journal of the History of the Neurosciences* 2010;19:195-198.

Papez JW, "Theodor Meynert." In: Haymaker W and Baer, Karl A, eds. *Founders of Neurology: One Hundred and Thirty-Three Biographical Sketches*. Springfield: Charles C. Thomas, 1953, pp. 64-67.

Pickles JO. Auditory pathways. In: *Handbook of Clinical Neurology*, v. 129 (3rd series), *The Human Auditory System* [eds. Celesia GG and Hickok G]. Amsterdam: Elsevier, 2015.

Raichle ME, Mintun MA. Brain work and brain imaging. *Annual Review of Neuroscience* 2006;29:449-476.

Satterthwaite TD, Davatzikos C. Towards an individualized delineation of functional neuroanatomy. *Neuron* 2015;87:471-473.

Schmahmann JD. From movement to thought: anatomic substrate of the cerebellar contribution to cognitive processing. *Human Brain Mapping* 1996;4:174-198.

Seitelberger F. Theodor Meynert (1833-1892): Pioneer and visionary of brain research. *Journal of the History of the Neurosciences* 1997;6(3):264-274.

Shoja MM. Tubbs RS, Loukas M, Shokouhi G, Ardalan MR. Marie-François Xaxier Bichat (1771-1802) and his contributions to the foundations of pathological anatomy and modern medicine. *Annals of Anatomy* 2008;190:413-420.

Stookey B. Jean-Baptiste Bouillaud and Ernest Auburtin: early studies on cerebral localization and the speech center. *Journal of the American Medical Association* 1963;184:1024-1029.

Van Essen DC, Maunsell JHR. Two-dimensional maps of the cerebral cortex. *Journal of Comparative Neurology* 1980;191:255-281.

Wernicke C. *Der Aphasische Symptomencomplex: Eine Psychologische Studie auf Anatomische Basis*. Breslau: Cohn, 1874. [I translated the original text and checked myself using Eggert, 1977 and the translation referenced as Wernicke, 1969.]

Wernicke C. The symptom complex of aphasia. A psychological study on an anatomical basis. In: *Boston Studies in the Philosophy of Science* (vol. IV), eds. Cohen, Robert S. and Wartofsky, Marx W. Dordrecht: D. Reidel Publishing, 1969, pp. 34-97.

Whitaker HA, Etlinger SC. Theodor Meynert's contribution to classical 19th century aphasia studies. *Brain and Language* 1993;45:560-571.

Williams JCP, Barratt-Boyes BG, Lowe JB. Supravalvular aortic stenosis. *Circulation* 1961;24:1311-1318.

Yates AJ. Delayed auditory feedback. *Psychological Bulletin* 1963;60(3):213-232.

www.ingramcontent.com/pod-product-compliance
Lightning Source LLC
Chambersburg PA
CBHW031925240526
45464CB00022B/877